Teen Health Series

Breastfeeding
SOURCEBOOK

Health Reference Series

First Edition

Breastfeeding
SOURCEBOOK

Basic Consumer Health Information about the Benefits of Breastmilk, Preparing to Breastfeed, Breastfeeding as a Baby Grows, Nutrition, and More, Including Information on Special Situations and Concerns Such as Mastitis, Illness, Medications, Allergies, Multiple Births, Prematurity, Special Needs, and Adoption

Along with a Glossary and Resources for Additional Help and Information

Edited by
Jenni Lynn Colson

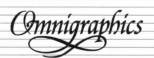

615 Griswold Street • Detroit, MI 48226

Bibliographic Note

Because this page cannot legibly accommodate all the copyright notices, the Bibliographic Note portion of the Preface constitutes an extension of the copyright notice.

Edited by Jenni Lynn Colson

Health Reference Series

Karen Bellenir, *Managing Editor*
David A. Cooke, MD, *Medical Consultant*
Elizabeth Barbour, *Permissions Associate*
Maria Franklin, *Permissions Assistant*
Joan Margeson, *Research Associate*
Dawn Matthews, *Verification Assistant*
Carol Munson, *Permissions Assistant*
Laura Pleva, *Index Editor*
EdIndex, Services for Publishers, *Indexers*

* * *

Omnigraphics, Inc.

Matthew P. Barbour, *Senior Vice President*
Kay Gill, *Vice President—Directories*
Kevin Hayes, *Operations Manager*
David P. Bianco, *Marketing Consultant*

* * *

Peter E. Ruffner, *President and Publisher*
Frederick G. Ruffner, Jr., *Chairman*
Copyright © 2002 Omnigraphics, Inc.
ISBN 0-7808-0332-9

Library of Congress Cataloging-in-Publication Data

Breastfeeding sourcebook : basic consumer health information about the benefits of breastmilk, preparing to breastfeed, breastfeeding as a baby grows, nutrition, and more, including information on special situations and concerns such as mastitis, illness, medications, allergies, multiple births, prematurity, special needs, and adoption; along with a glossary and resources for additional help and information / edited by Jenni Lynn Colson.-- 1st ed.
    p. cm.-- (Health reference series)
  Includes index
  ISBN 0-7808-0332-9 (lib. bdg. : alk. paper)
    1. Breast feeding. 2. Consumer education. I. Colson, Jenni Lynn. II. Health reference series (Unnumbered)
RJ216 .B7798 2002
649'.33--dc21
2002023316

Printed in the United States

Table of Contents

Part VI: Breastfeeding and the Working Mother

Part VII: Special Situations

Part VIII: Additional Help and Information

Preface

About This Book

Experts agree that breastmilk is the ideal nutrition for a healthy, full-term baby and is the only food needed for the first six months of life. Besides its nutritional value, breastmilk provides protection against diseases, infections, and allergies; benefits brain development; and continually changes to meet a growing baby's needs. Human milk contains at least 100 ingredients not found in infant formula, and even infant formula manufacturers agree that breastmilk is best for babies. However, only half of all babies in the United States are breastfed, and less than twenty percent are still breastfeeding by age six months.

This *Sourcebook* contains basic consumer health information about the benefits of breastmilk; the basics of breastmilk production; and tips on overcoming common challenges that breastfeeding families face, including breast troubles, allergies, colic, and illness. It offers tips for breastfeeding babies from birth to weaning; tells when and how to find support; and addresses special situations like multiple births, adoption, special needs, prematurity, and working mothers. A glossary and resources for additional help and information are also included.

How to Use This Book

This book is divided into parts and chapters. Parts focus on broad areas of interest. Chapters are devoted to single topics within a part.

Part I: Why Breastfeed? explains the many ways in which breast-feeding benefits babies, mothers, and the environment. It debunks commonly held myths about breastfeeding and explores factors influencing a woman's decision to breastfeed.

Part II: Preparing to Breastfeed examines who breastfeeds, offers an overview of the breastfeeding process, and explains how human milk is produced. Parents are provided with information about choosing a doctor who is supportive of breastfeeding and other steps in planning for a successful breastfeeding experience.

Part III: Breastfeeding in the Early Weeks explains what parents, doctors, and hospitals can do to contribute to a successful breastfeeding experience in the early weeks. It also offers mothers information on caring for themselves after the birth process and for dealing with postpartum depression.

Part IV: Breastfeeding as a Baby Grows addresses common concerns parents of breastfeeding babies may have, including how to be sure a baby is getting enough milk, using bottles, introducing solids, and weaning. Three final chapters offer information for parents about nutrition for the nursing mother, birth control, and how fathers can support breastfeeding.

Part V: Breastfeeding Difficulties explores some of the challenges that may arise while breastfeeding and offers suggestions for overcoming these challenges which include soreness, reduced milk supply, colic, allergies, thrush, and nursing strikes. A final section focuses on how and when to seek help from a lactation professional.

Part VI: Breastfeeding and Returning to Work addresses the special issues faced by mothers who return to work and continue to breastfeed. This section includes suggestions for communicating with employers, selecting and using a breastpump, and safely storing breastmilk.

Part VII: Special Situations focuses on birth, medical, and other issues that affect the breastfeeding relationship, including premature, multiple, and cesearean births, babies with special needs, and breastfeeding the adopted baby. Information is also provided for teen mothers, as well as mothers with cancer, lupus, and HIV/AIDS. A final chapter explains situations in which a mother should not breastfeed.

Part VIII: Additional Help and Information contains medication precautions for breastfeeding mothers, an outline of government initiatives to increase breastfeeding rates, and an overview of legal issues related to breastfeeding. A glossary of terms is provided, as well as resources for breastfeeding organizations, information, and products.

Bibliographic Note

This volume contains documents and excerpts from publications issued by the following government agencies: Center for Disease Control and Prevention (CDC), National Institues of Health (NIH), National Institute of Child Health and Human Development (NICHD), U.S. Agency for International Development (USAID), U.S. Department of Health and Human Services Office on Women's Health, U.S. Department of Agriculture, and the U.S. Food and Drug Administration.

This volume also contains copyrighted documents produced by the following organizations and individuals: Academy for Educational Development, American Academy of Family Physicians, Baylor College of Medicine, Breastfeeding.com, Breastfeeding Task Force of Greater Los Angeles, Dr. Jack Newman, Family Collection, King County Washington Public Health Department, La Leche League International (LLLI), Lactation Education Resources On-Line (LERON), Medical Reporter, Medicinenet.com, Micromedex, Inc., Promotion of Mother's Milk (ProMoM, Inc.), San Diego County Breastfeeding Coalition, University Hospitals of Cleveland, University of Iowa, University of Rhode Island Cooperative Extension, University of Texas Southwestern Medical Center, and WideSmiles.

Full citation information is provided on the first page of each chapter. Every effort has been made to secure all necessary rights to reprint the copyrighted material. If any omissions have been made, please contact Omnigraphics to make corrections for future editions.

Acknowledgements

A special thank you to Karen Bellenir for her continous support and guidance. Thanks also go to Maria Franklin, Carol Munson, Dawn Matthews, and Dr. David Cooke for their assistance with this book.

Note from the Editor

This book is part of Omnigraphics' *Health Reference Series*. The series provides basic information about a broad range of medical concerns. It is not intended to serve as a tool for diagnosing illness, in prescribing treatments, or as a substitute for the physician/patient relationship. All persons concerned about medical symptoms or the possibility of disease are encouraged to seek professional care from an appropriate health care provider.

Our Advisory Board

The *Health Reference Series* is reviewed by an Advisory Board comprised of librarians from public, academic, and medical libraries. We would like to thank the following board members for providing guidance to the development of this series:

Dr. Lynda Baker, Associate Professor of Library and Information Science, Wayne State University, Detroit, MI

Nancy Bulgarelli, William Beaumont Hospital Library, Royal Oak, MI

Karen Imarisio, Bloomfield Township Public Library, Bloomfield Township, MI

Karen Morgan, Mardigian Library, University of Michigan-Dearborn, Dearborn, MI

Rosemary Orlando, St. Clair Shores Public Library, St. Clair Shores, MI

Medical Consultant

Medical consultation services are provided to the *Health Reference Series* editors by David A. Cooke, M.D. Dr. Cooke is a graduate of Brandeis University, and he received his M.D. degree from the University of Michigan. He completed residency training at the University of Wisconsin Hospital and Clinics and is board-certified in Internal Medicine. Dr. Cooke currently works as part of the University of Michigan Health System and practices in Brighton, MI. In his free time, he enjoys writing, science fiction, and spending time with his family.

Health Reference Series *Update Policy*

The inaugural book in the *Health Reference Series* was the first edition of *Cancer Sourcebook* published in 1992. Since then, the *Series* has been enthusiastically received by librarians and in the medical community. In order to maintain the standard of providing high-quality health information for the layperson the editorial staff at Omnigraphics felt it was necessary to implement a policy of updating volumes when warranted.

Medical researchers have been making tremendous strides, and it is the purpose of the *Health Reference Series* to stay current with the most recent advances. Each decision to update a volume will be made on an individual basis. Some of the considerations will include how much new information is available and the feedback we receive from people who use the books. If there is a topic you would like to see added to the update list, or an area of medical concern you feel has not been adequately addressed, please write to:

Editor
Health Reference Series
Omnigraphics, Inc.
615 Griswold
Detroit, MI 48226

The commitment to providing on-going coverage of important medical developments has also led to some format changes in the *Health Reference Series*. Each new volume on a topic is individually titled and called a "First Edition." Subsequent updates will carry sequential edition numbers. To help avoid confusion and to provide maximum flexibility in our ability to respond to informational needs, the practice of consecutively numbering each volume has been discontinued.

Part One

Why Breastfeed?

Chapter 1

Breastfeeding: Good for Babies, Mothers, and the Planet

Good for Babies

Human Milk's Nutritional Benefits

Human milk, the best food for babies, contains the right amount of nutrients, in the right proportions, for the growing baby. A living, biological fluid, it contains many unique components. For example, lactoferrin provides optimal absorption of iron and protects the gut from harmful bacteria, lipases assist in digestion of fats, and special growth factors and hormones contribute to optimal growth and development. A mother's own milk changes during a feeding from thirst quenching to hunger satisfying, and comes in a variety of flavors as a mother's diet varies. Its composition changes as the baby grows to meet baby's changing nutritional needs. It serves as the nutritional model for artificial baby milks, but none of these can match it.

While most people are aware that human milk provides excellent nutrition, many people are unaware of breastfeeding's other health benefits for babies.

Breastfeeding and the Immune System

Human milk is a baby's first immunization. It provides antibodies which protect baby from many common respiratory and intestinal

Excerpted from "If Breastfeeding Is So Wonderful, Why Aren't More Women Doing It?" by Alicia Dermer, M.D., I.B.C.L.C. © 1998-2000 by Joel R. Cooper, *The Medical Reporter*, http://medicalreporter.health.org. Used with permission.

diseases, and also contains living immune cells. First milk, colostrum, is packed with components which increase immunity and protect the newborn's intestines. Artificially fed babies have higher rates of middle ear infections, pneumonia, and cases of gastroenteritis (stomach flu). Breastfeeding as an infant also provides protection from developing immune system cancers such as lymphoma, bowel diseases such as Crohn's disease and celiac sprue, and juvenile rheumatoid arthritis, all of which are related to immune system function. Breastfed babies generally mount a more effective response to childhood immunizations. In all these cases, benefits begin immediately, and increase with increasing duration of breastfeeding.

Babies from families with a tendency to allergic diseases particularly benefit from breastfeeding. Exclusive breastfeeding, especially if it continues for at least six months, provides protection against allergies, asthma, and eczema.

Infant Growth and Development

New growth charts from the World Health Organization confirm that breastfed infants grow differently from formula fed babies. Breastfed infants grow faster initially, then slow down as they approach their first birthday. This can sometimes be interpreted as "dropping off the growth curve," but really represents normal growth. People artificially fed as infants go on to have a higher risk of obesity as adults.

More and more research is showing that breastfeeding leads to optimal brain development. While there are behavioral aspects to this, the milk is important, too. One study of premature babies who were tube-fed breastmilk or artificial milk, but were never breastfed directly, showed that the babies who received no breas milk had IQs 8 points lower on average than those who received breastmilk. Human milk has special ingredients like DHA (docosohexaenoic acid) and AA (arachidonic acid) which contribute to brain and retinal development. And all breastfed babies tend to spend a lot of their time in the "quiet alert" state which is most conducive to learning.

Breastfeeding in Special Circumstances

Breastfeeding has other special benefits for premature infants. Premature breastmilk contains different amounts of some nutrients than term breastmilk, which are more suited to the needs of premature babies. Necrotizing enterocolitis, a serious bowel inflammation, is very rare for breastfed infants. And of course they get the same immune protection, which may be even more critical for premature babies, and has been shown to reduce the risk of sepsis in these babies. Suckling at the breast, and digesting breastmilk, cause less stress for the premature infant than bottle-feeding does; so most premature babies can go to breast as soon as they are able to suckle. Because of the reduction in infections and the shorter time to full feeding, breastfed premature infants can usually leave the neonatal intensive care unit (NICU) sooner. For some babies, breastfeeding is a life-and-death matter. In addition to its known benefit where water supplies are unsafe or food supplies erratic, breastfeeding lowers the risk of SIDS in all populations.

There are very few reasons, particularly from the baby's point of view, to avoid breastfeeding. Most authorities recommend that US mothers who are HIV positive not breastfeed; however, in many areas of the world breastfeeding's known benefits outweigh the small risk of transmission from breastmilk. Few other medical conditions preclude breastfeeding, as there are many appropriate medications that are suitable for use in breastfeeding moms.

Breastfeeding's immunologic and developmental benefits may be particularly important for babies with medical problems such as congenital heart disease, cleft palate, Down's syndrome, etc. In cases where the baby has a problem which affects ability to suckle at the breast, expressed breastmilk from mother is still the best choice. Banked human milk, the availability of which is unfortunately limited, would be the second choice. Commercial artificial baby milks are preferable to other alternatives, but far from perfect substitutes for human milk. For every "new" component that is added to commercial baby milks to make them closer to human milk, several more components of human milk are discovered.

It's Not JUST the Milk, Either!

In addition to all the known benefits of human milk, it's also clear that the act of breastfeeding is beneficial. Breastfeeding's contribution to optimal oral development means less risk of malocclusion—and perhaps lower orthodontist bills! Bottle-fed babies have a higher risk of baby bottle tooth decay, as well. Close skin-to-skin contact with mother provides optimal nurturing and an almost automatic close emotional attachment. Suckling at breast optimizes hand-to-eye coordination, especially with regular "side-switching." Even in the rare cases when mother can't produce enough milk, or for adopted babies, supplemental systems can allow mother and baby to enjoy a breastfeeding relationship.

Good for Mothers

The extent to which breastfeeding affects mothers' health is rarely emphasized. Much of the lay literature about breastfeeding makes it sound like a rather time-consuming, difficult, and even painful experience that women must endure for the sake of their babies' health. No wonder some mothers are left with the impression that they must "martyr" themselves and breastfeed for their baby's sake.

Surprise: Breastfeeding is good for mothers, too! Not only that, but it is a joyful, relaxing experience. Although breastfeeding advocates have been criticized for oversimplifying and not informing mothers of potential problems of breastfeeding, the truth of the matter is that when practiced optimally breastfeeding is an enjoyable experience, pure and simple. We must remember that many of the problems and inconveniences so commonly described in the lay literature and passed around by word of mouth as "horror stories" are due to the fact that we live in a bottle-feeding society, with little family or social support and little understanding of breastfeeding by many health care professionals. Thus, problems such as "insufficient milk syndrome," engorgement, cracked and bleeding nipples, all of which would be rare in a breastfeeding society, have become commonplace.

Physical Health Benefits for Mothers

First of all, it almost goes without saying, but what's good for babies is good for mothers. In other words, healthier babies are less stressful to care for, and the decreased medical costs are a boon to the family. Furthermore, the optimal neurological and intellectual development provide potential long-term benefits to the family.

In addition, there are many direct health benefits to breastfeeding mothers. Immediately after birth, repeated bursts of oxytocin released in response to the baby's sucking cause contraction of the uterus. This protects mothers from postpartum hemorrhage (bottle-feeding mothers get oxytocin intravenously immediately after birth, but for the next 24–48 hours during which risk of hemorrhage is highest, they're on their own). Continued exclusive nursing (i.e., breastfeeding without added bottles of formula or solids) tends to delay the return of ovulation and menstruation. In fact, the lactational amenorrhea method (LAM) is a well-studied method of child spacing which is 99% effective in preventing pregnancy in the first six months as long as exclusive nursing is practiced. For mothers who don't practice exclusive breastfeeding, there is still some relative protection; and most contraceptives including barrier methods, IUD's, and even progesterone-only hormonal contraceptives such as the "mini-pill" or injectable "depo" progesterone, are all compatible with breastfeeding. There's no need to stop breastfeeding in order to use effective birth control.

In addition to the child-spacing advantage, the delayed menses also decrease the mother's iron losses. When combined with improved iron absorption from the gut, the net effect (despite some iron use for breastmilk production) is decreased risk of iron deficiency anemia.

Another well-documented benefit of breastfeeding is more rapid and sustained weight loss. Milk production uses up 200–500 calories a day. To burn off an equivalent number of calories, a bottle-feeding mother would need to swim 30 laps or ride a bicycle for over an hour. In our opinion, breastfeeding is definitely easier! Mothers who have had gestational diabetes benefit particularly from the efficient use of calories during breastfeeding, since a return to optimal weight may prevent subsequent development of diabetes. Furthermore, diabetic mothers who breastfeed tend to need less insulin or medication for their diabetes.

The prolonged suppression of ovulatory cycles appears to be associated with significant long-term health advantages as well. Mothers who breastfeed for at least 6 months throughout their lifetime have a decreased risk of breast cancer, and similar reduced rates have been shown for ovarian and uterine cancers. Even being breastfed has been associated with decreased risk of breast cancer, over and above the fact that women who were breastfed themselves are more likely to breastfeed their own children.

For some time, there was concern about calcium loss during lactation and potential for osteoporosis. In fact, some literature actually lists breastfeeding as a risk factor for osteoporosis. Current medical literature demonstrates that not only is the loss in bone density during breastfeeding temporary, reverting to normal after weaning, but that bones may actually be stronger after prolonged breastfeeding. Far from a risk factor for osteoporosis, breastfeeding may actually protect against it.

The impact of breastfeeding on other women's illnesses needs further study. One example is the connection between breastfeeding and cholesterol levels. Breastfeeding mothers tend to have high total cholesterol levels, made up largely of the HDL ("good") fraction. This may prove to decrease the risk of coronary artery disease.

Are there any known harmful effects of breastfeeding on women's health? A couple of studies have demonstrated an increased risk of rheumatoid arthritis flare-ups and increased severity of arthritis in nursing mothers. Whether it is breastfeeding or some other confounding factor which causes this increase remains to be determined.

Psychosocial Issues in Breastfeeding and Women's Health

What about the emotional aspect of women's health? Where does breastfeeding fit in? Let's talk about mother-infant bonding, a somewhat controversial subject. Much is made about the way that breastfeeding facilitates this bonding, while at the same time it is clear that bottle-feeding mothers usually establish deep emotional bonds with their babies. This issue is difficult to study scientifically, but there is evidence of hormonal effects of breastfeeding which may predispose a mother to closer bonding with her infant. Combined with the automatic skin-to-skin contact and closeness afforded by breastfeeding (something which bottle-feeding mothers have to work to duplicate), this could result in improved bonding. An interesting sideline from a study in a developing country found that when breastfeeding rates were increased among mothers with a significant abandonment rate, fewer of these mothers abandoned their babies. Other studies have suggested that there may be a lower rate of child abuse in breastfeeding families considered to be at risk.

Another common psychological issue after birth is postpartum depression (PPD). The role of breastfeeding in this area is not clear, with some studies showing increased rates of PPD among breastfeeding mothers, others lower rates. The cause of PPD is unknown, and is probably due to a number of factors, including hormonal changes and lack of support in the new overwhelming role of motherhood. For some depressed mothers, their breastfeeding relationship takes on special importance. Sometimes, when antidepressant medications are deemed necessary, doctors are concerned about prescribing them for a breastfeeding mother. Antidepressants have been studied, and some have been demonstrated not to get to the baby or cause any symptoms. The small potential risk of the medication to the baby has to be weighed against the potential emotional devastation to an already depressed mother of having to wean her baby, as well as the known detrimental effects on infant emotional development when mother suffers from persistent depression.

Let's consider the situation of mothers who need to return to work. Is it worth it to breastfeed at all? Is it necessary to wean the baby when returning to work? Is pumping and storing mother's milk worth the effort? The answer to these questions is: yes, no, and definitely. Even if a mother needs to return to work within weeks and will be unable to pump while at work, the baby benefits from the colostrum and early milk and mother gets the experience of the closeness and bonding. On return to work a breastfeeding mother has three options:

- continue to breastfeed exclusively by nursing while at home and pumping her milk while at work,

- continue to nurse while at home and feed formula while at work, or

- wean completely to formula.

Clearly, any amount of continued breastfeeding would be preferable to weaning. Studies have shown that babies in day care whose mothers provide their milk have the fewest days out of day care and their mothers have the fewest missed days from work, while those who were breastfed and got some formula were sick more often. The mothers of completely formula-fed babies had the most days out of work to care for their sick babies.

Although pumping and storing may sound daunting and time consuming, most mothers whose employers give breastfeeding support find that they work into an easy routine, and the work of pumping is worth it for the peace of mind of a healthier child and the continued bonding from breastfeeding on returning home. Increasing numbers of companies, in response to studies showing economic benefits, are instituting policies supportive of continued breastfeeding for their employees. Additionally, the cost of renting or even purchasing a pump is much lower than the cost of formula.

Breastfeeding and Fathers

So what's in it for Dad? Breastfeeding benefits fathers, too. First, and most straightforward, breastfed babies have less offensive dirty diapers. There are no bottles to prepare and warm in the middle of the night. Fathers benefit from having a healthy baby; and can play with, snuggle, and bathe the baby as their relationship develops. If participating in feeding is important, he can be the main solid-food feeder later. Dads generally also appreciate the impact on the family budget of lower health care costs, fewer sick days, and lack of need to buy formula. And all of the health benefits for mothers make it likely that his partner will be healthier.

Good for the Environment

Another important issue related to infant feeding and health is the interaction between infant feeding method and the environment. Breastfeeding is a completely natural, efficient use of resources. In contrast, artificial feeding involves:

- overgrazing of land by cattle;
- use of chemical fertilizers to grow the soy;
- use of valuable environmental resources for formula production;
- packaging and transportation of the product;
- use of water and fuel for mixing and heating the product and for sterilizing bottles and nipples;
- waste disposal of the cans, bottles, accessories, cartons, etc.

Despite this, the media and some environmental groups tend to play up issues of environmental contaminants in mother's milk. In fact, except in situations of toxic spills or occupational exposure to hazardous levels, breastfeeding has caused no ill effects in babies. To the contrary, studies comparing breastfed and bottle-fed babies in the same environment have shown better development and less cancer in the breastfed babies.

Furthermore, despite concerns about PCBs in breastmilk potentially producing infertility in the offspring, the major burden of PCBs gets to babies during pregnancy. In addition, cows get exposed to PCBs, too, so artificial milks are not necessarily "pure," either. A lesser known and less publicized issue is the fact that soy formulas contain phytoestrogens, which may have just as serious long-term effects. Rather than calling for women to avoid breastfeeding, the call needs to be to continue to clean up the environment to safeguard everyone's health. Breastfeeding will contribute to this cleanup effort.

Conclusion

In light of the overwhelming evidence of breastfeeding benefits not only for babies but also for mothers and the planet, it seems fair to say that the choice of an infant feeding method is far more than the choice between two relatively similar methods with only convenience as the deciding factor. When a mother chooses not to breastfeed or decides to wean early from the breast, she is not merely substituting an inferior artificial substance without any disease-protection properties for her child and feeding her child with an unnatural implement. She is also potentially affecting her own immediate and long-term health in many ways. Artificial feeding increases personal and societal health care costs and detrimentally affects the environment.

Breastfeeding in a society where bottle-feeding is the norm clearly requires a significant commitment, especially when relatives and friends do not support breastfeeding. However, women making the decision about infant feeding should know that breastfeeding is clearly more than a lifestyle choice: it is a significant health decision with lifelong consequences.

Chapter 2

Risks of Formula Feeding

The practice of feeding babies infant formula, rather than breastmilk, carries with it profound risks in modern, industrialized countries, as well as in developing countries. While many are familiar with the well-publicized tragedies of formula-fed infants in developing countries, many are unaware of how the lack of breastmilk and the use of infant formula compromise the health and well being of children in the United States. These risks are well documented in the medical literature. A few are listed below.

Illness and Hospitalization

- Formula feeding accounts for up to 26% of insulin dependent diabetes mellitus in children.

- Otitis media (middle ear infection) is up to 3–4 times as prevalent in formula-fed infants.

- US formula-fed infants have a ten-fold risk of being hospitalized for any bacterial infection.

"The Risks of Infant Formula Feeding," undated. Reprinted with permission of the Breastfeeding Task Force of Greater Los Angeles, 12781 Schabarum Avenue, Irwindale, CA 91706; Telephone: 626-856-6650, Internet: www.BreastfeedingTask ForLA.org.

Mortality

- One sudden infant death for every 1000 live birth occurs as a result of failure to breastfeed in western industrialized nations.

- For every 1000 babies born in the US each year, four die because they are not breastfed.

Development and Intelligence

- Scores on the Baley Mental Development Index were lower in formula-fed children at 1–2 years of age. Scores were directly correlated with the duration of breastfeeding.

- Formula-fed pre-term infants had lower IQ scores (8 points) at age 7–8 years than breastfed preemies, even after adjustment for mother's education and social class.

Composition and Contamination of Infant Formula

- Due to an excessive phosphate load in formula, formula fed infants face a thirty-fold risk of neonatal hypocalcemic tetany (convulsions, seizures, twitching) during the first ten days of life.

- Formula fed infants are at a high risk of exposure to life-threatening bacterial contamination. *Enterobacter sakazakii* is a frequent contaminant in powdered formula and can cause sepsis and meningitis in newborns.

Specific references available upon request. An excellent source of additional information can be found in *Breastfeeding: A Guide for the Medical Profession*, 1999 (5th Ed) Ruth A. Lawrence and Robert M. Lawrence, MD Mosby Year Book.

Chapter 3

If Breastfeeding Is So Great, Why Are the Rates So Low?

Baby-Unfriendly Hospital Practices

Hospital practices contribute to widespread breastfeeding failure. The routine use of drugs during labor and delivery often results in babies arriving in this world in a drugged state, unable to latch onto the breast. The immediate separation of mother and baby so that the baby can undergo routine tests and procedures (all of which could be delayed without any harm to the baby) also interferes with the baby's ability to initiate breastfeeding during the crucial first hour after birth, when most babies are in a relaxed, alert, and receptive state. Unnecessarily aggressive suctioning of the airway immediately after birth traumatizes some babies so much that they shy away from all oral stimuli—including bottles—for days after birth. Many babies are routinely given bottles of formula or glucose water in the hospital nursery, even when their mothers have requested that no bottles be given and that their babies be brought to them to nurse. Since formula is easier to get out of a bottle than human milk is from the breast, even one bottle feeding can cause some babies to form an irreversible preference (sometimes known as "nipple confusion") for the bottle nipple; those babies may never be able to breastfeed normally.

Formula Company Marketing Practices

Formula marketing targets women. New mothers are given free samples of formula, babies are given bottles in hospitals, coupons or food samples arrive in the mail, and booklets and videotapes are distributed on breastfeeding and weaning. The World Health Organization's Code for the Marketing of Breastmilk Substitutes prohibits marketing of these products in these ways. It covers formula, other milk products, cereals, teas, and juices; as well as bottles and nipples. The Code has ten important provisions.

1. NO advertising of any of these products to the public.

2. NO free samples to mothers.

3. NO promotion of products in health care facilities, including the distribution of free or low-cost supplies.

4. NO company sales representatives to advise mothers.

5. NO gifts or personal samples to health workers.

6. NO words or pictures idealizing artificial feeding, or pictures of infants on labels of infant milk containers.

7. Information to health workers should be scientific and factual.

8. ALL information on artificial infant feeding, including that on labels, should explain the benefits of breastfeeding and the costs and hazards associated with artificial feeding.

9. Unsuitable products, such as sweetened condensed milk, should not be promoted for babies.

10. Manufacturers and distributors should comply with the Code's provisions even if countries have not adopted laws or other measures.

Imagine what it would be like if breastfeeding were advertised competitively with formula!

Medical Professionals Lack Knowledge about Breastfeeding

Another related reason for low breastfeeding rates is the almost complete absence of breastfeeding curricula in medical schools. A study published in the *Journal of the American Medical Association* shows that most doctors know little about breastfeeding. (Freed GL et al: National assessment of physicians' breast-feeding knowledge, attitudes, training, and experience. *JAMA* 1995;273:472-476). The study looked at doctors' knowledge of the clinical aspects of breastfeeding. It revealed disturbingly high rates of ignorance about why breastfeeding is important and how to handle breastfeeding difficulties. The authors of this study surveyed more than 3,000 residents and nearly 2,000 physicians practicing obstetrics, pediatrics, and family medicine and found that few of them knew the basics of breastfeeding such as how to teach a new mother to use a breast pump or what to do about low milk supply. Many doctors who are not educated about breastfeeding advise supplementing with formula when any problem arises with breastfeeding. The result: the baby is quickly weaned from the breast to the bottle because the mother's milk supply diminishes immediately in response to her baby's diminishing demand for her milk.

Interestingly, the study found that most important factor influencing whether a physician was knowledgeable about breastfeeding was whether the doctor herself, or the doctor's wife, had breastfed children.

The Bottle-Feeding Culture

Another big reason for the low breastfeeding rates is the bottle-feeding culture that has developed as a result of formula promotion and medical ignorance of breastfeeding. Babies are associated closely with bottles, not breasts. Go to any toy store. It is difficult to find a baby doll that doesn't come with a bottle. Look around you where mothers with babies can be found. Most of the babies are fed with bottles. The sight of a woman breastfeeding her child in public is so rare as to be remarkable.

The result is that the chain of cultural breastfeeding knowledge has been broken. Where breastfeeding is the norm, girls grow up seeing their mothers breastfeeding their younger siblings, their aunts breastfeeding their cousins, their older sisters breastfeeding their nieces and nephews, their neighbors breastfeeding their children, etc. Breastfeeding is a normal part of everyday life, and a girl inherits the accumulated knowledge of previous generations about such things as how to position the baby at the breast, how to tell if you have a letdown of the milk, and how to tell if the baby is properly latched on and is getting milk.

New mothers in a bottle-feeding culture need expert medical advice to take the place of the lost cultural knowledge of breastfeeding. As the study cited above makes clear, such advice is unlikely to come from your doctor. Someone with specific training in human lactation, such as a board certified lactation consultant or a leader from a mother-to-mother support group (like La Leche League International) is much more likely to be able to help you with breastfeeding problems.

Maternal Employment

The belief that breastfeeding cannot continue when the mother works is an unfortunate misconception. An employer need only make minor accommodations to allow employees to breastfeed their babies. With a clean, private place and about 20 minutes every 4 hours, a mother can express her milk for later use by her baby. With on-site or nearby daycare, a mother can breastfeed her baby directly during brief breaks. Even a mother who cannot pump or breastfeed during the workday can breastfeed her baby when they are together and supplement with formula at other times.

Chapter 4

Breastfeeding Myths and Realities

Myth 1: Breastfeeding Ruins the Shape of Your Breasts

Reality: This is simply not true. As soon as a woman becomes pregnant permanent changes occur in her breasts. Even if she doesn't carry to term, or chooses to abort, her breasts will never be the same as they were before she became pregnant. Whether or not she then goes on to breastfeed will not effect her future breast shape one way or another. Heredity plays a large role in this matter, as does excessive weight gain or loss. It is helpful to maintain the tone of the muscles that support your breasts, and to avoid large and sudden weight gains or losses (pregnancy related or otherwise).

Myth 2: Small-Breasted Women Won't Have Enough Milk

Reality: The size of your breasts, either large or small, has nothing to do with the amount of milk they will produce. Almost all women who are getting plenty of liquid, adequate rest and relaxation, and lots of physical contact with their babies will produce enough milk. In fact, many women who believe they are not producing enough milk are mistaken. It is surprising how much milk a tiny baby can consume in a short amount of time. The number of wet and soiled diapers being produced every day is a fairly accurate indicator of how

Leslie Kincaid Burby, ©1998, Promotion of Mothers' Milk (ProMoM, Inc.), www.ProMoM.org. Reprinted with permission.

19

much milk the baby is getting. Six–eight wet cloth diapers (5–6 soaked disposables), and at least 2–5 bowel movements per day indicate that your baby is getting plenty of milk. Once the newborn stage is over, the number of bowel movements may decrease.

If your baby seems lethargic, seems to have poor skin tone, or is not wetting and soiling an adequate number of diapers, this is cause for concern. If you believe you are having trouble with your milk supply, contact a lactation consultant or a supportive physician. It is always better to be safe than sorry.

Remember, the more the baby nurses, the more milk your breasts will be stimulated to produce. If you begin "supplementing" your supply with artificial milk, your breasts will not receive adequate stimulation and your milk supply will decrease.

Myth 3: Breastfeeding Influences a Baby's Future Sexual Orientation

Reality: Not true. The misconception that breastfeeding could in some way determine whether a child will grow up to be heterosexual or homosexual is tied to the mistaken idea that breastfeeding is in itself a sort of sexual activity. It is not. Breastfeeding is a nutritional and nurturing act that helps children grow up to be healthier and more self confident, whatever their sexual preference turns out to be.

Myth 4: Today's Artificial Breastmilk Is Just as Good as the Real Thing

Reality: Even though modern formulas are considerably better than some of the old fashioned ones, they can never replicate mother's milk. In the first place, human milk contains live cells and human hormones that are impossible to obtain from the milk of another species. Furthermore, formula companies admit that they don't yet know all of the ingredients in human breastmilk. Every few months these companies come up with something different to try to add in. If you choose to breastfeed you can be confident that all the necessary nutrients, immunities, hormones, and as yet undiscovered beneficial elements will be present in the right amounts. On the other hand, research shows significant risk in the use of artificial milk.

Myth 5: Breastfeeding Takes More Time than Bottle-Feeding

Reality: This statement is usually made in reference to night feedings. If a mother sleeps with or next to her baby, night feedings are much easier than they are for bottle-fed babies. All she has to do is open her nightgown and roll over. Even if the breastfeeding mother does not sleep with her baby, it is certainly less time consuming to go pick up the child and offer the breast than to get up, go the kitchen, open a can of formula (or mix up a batch from powder), turn on the stove to boil water to heat the formula, put the formula into a bottle, warm the bottle in the hot water, wait several minutes, return to the crying child, pick up the child, and offer the bottle. Of course, at this point it is tempting for an exhausted mother or father to prop up the bottle and leave the baby alone to finish it. This is an extremely dangerous thing to do as the baby can easily choke on the liquid, or spit up and choke. Also, it leads to baby bottle tooth decay.

It is true that you may have to feed a bit more frequently if you breastfeed because breastmilk is more easily digested than formula. Of course that easy digestibility translates into less time dealing with colic, diarrhea, and other digestive ailments. Also, breastfed babies are far less likely to contract colds, ear infections, and asthma. Formula-feeding mothers need to factor in extra time for trips to the store to buy supplies, as well as possible extra trips to the doctor's office.

It is also a fact that in the early months, unless you express breastmilk, you will be the only person able to provide nutrition to your baby. Formula-feeding mothers can have other caregivers give some or most of the feedings. However, breastfeeding offers a new mother an amazing chance to bond with her child, as well as all the health benefits that formula and bottles cannot provide. It may be helpful to remember that your baby will only be completely dependent on you for a very short amount of time in the course of your relationship together. Nursing can give you a chance for a much needed relaxation break, and time to reconnect with your baby. Try to savor these special moments.

Myth 6: You Can't Get Pregnant If You're Breastfeeding

Reality: True and false! Breastfeeding is only an effective form of birth control (98%) during the first six months, and is only effective during this period if the baby is receiving nothing but breastmilk on demand. No supplements, no solids, no water, and no pacifiers! The chance of pregnancy increases greatly when the baby begins sleeping through the night, starts eating solids, and/or when the mother resumes her menstrual cycle. If you truly do not wish to become pregnant again yet, it is wise to use an additional method of birth control.

Myth 7: You Must Wean If You Get Pregnant

Reality: There is no particular reason why a woman who is enjoying breastfeeding one child should wean that child when she learns that she is expecting another, unless she has a history of preterm labor. Some women continue to breastfeed throughout a pregnancy and then go on to "tandem" feed. This phrase refers to the practice of breastfeeding more than one child simultaneously. Some children do wean themselves once their mother becomes pregnant, possibly because her milk supply drops, or they detect a change in the taste of the milk which does not please them. Some women choose to wean because they find breastfeeding during pregnancy too physically or emotionally fatiguing. Other women describe enjoying the relaxation breaks that an ongoing breastfeeding process requires of them, and feel it contributes to the enjoyment of their new pregnancy. See La Leche League's information on breastfeeding during pregnancy.

Myth 8: You Can't Breastfeed after a Cesarean Section Birth

Reality: It is entirely possible to breastfeed after a c-section. Many women describe really enjoying being able to perform this natural act after going through a very medically oriented birth. It is important to nurse in way that does not put pressure on the incision sight. The football-hold position is particularly helpful, as is a good nursing pillow. Ask the hospital staff for help, and consider calling a lactation consultant or your local La Leche League if you're having difficulty.

Myth 9: Your Milk Will "Come in" Immediately after You Give Birth

Reality: First of all, the substance produced by your breasts immediately after a birth is called colostrum. It is yellowish and stickier than mature milk, and full of nutrients and immunities for the newborn baby. However, amounts of colostrum vary from mother to mother, and you may not produce very much. This is normal.

After colostrum the breast then begins to produce transitional milk, which is whitish-yellow, and more abundant. Gradually, over the next week or two, the transitional milk begins to change to a thin, bluish-white mature milk. Your milk production is directly linked to how often and how effectively your baby is suckling. If your transitional milk does not come in after 30–40 hours it is a good idea to contact a lactation consultant or La Leche League, especially if the hospital staff is advising you to give formula or water.

Myth 10: Your Mate Will Find You Less Attractive If You Breastfeed

Reality: It is possible that your mate may have some trouble adjusting to thinking of your breasts as sources of nourishment as well as of sexual stimulation. On the other hand, many partners find that a woman who is fulfilling this new part of her womanly potential is particularly exciting. If your mate does feel uncomfortable with this, however, it may be helpful to join a support group with other couples so that he/she may become more familiar with these new images, and begin to understand that they are normal and healthy.

Myth 11: Breastfeeding Is Painful

Reality: Many women experience no pain or difficulty at all when they start breastfeeding. For some, the first week or two may include some slight discomfort and pain. However, excruciating or ongoing pain is not normal. Usually, it is caused by incorrect positioning or latch-on technique, and can be cleared up with one or two visits from a lactation consultant. This pain can often be avoided if the mother does some reading, and/or attends a class about breastfeeding.

Visiting several La Leche League meetings while you are still pregnant is also a wonderful way to observe successfully breastfeeding mothers, as well as to network with other new parents. La Leche League has a peer counseling program in which you can receive help from other experienced mothers in the early days of your nursing relationship.

Do request any assistance you can from trained hospital staff while you are still in recovery. Sometimes these services are not volunteered, and you will not receive them unless you request them. Also, ask about the availability of a lactation consultant before you make your choice as to which hospital or birthing center you are planning to use.

Myth 12: You Can Be Arrested for Breastfeeding in Public

Reality: In the United States, you cannot be arrested for breast-feeding your child any place a woman would normally be. Such places include beaches, pools, restaurants (at the table), park benches, and parking lots, among others. You cannot be forced to remove yourself to a bathroom, closet, or vehicle. If anyone tries to tell you otherwise, you should feel free to refuse to comply, and inform them of your rights. Obviously, places like the men's bathrooms are off limits, since it's not a place women are supposed to be. Who would want to breastfeed there anyway?

Myth 13: You Can't Breastfeed If You Plan to Go Back to Work or School

Reality: If you're planning to return to work or school, there are several different ways to approach the situation without weaning your child. First of all, it may be possible to schedule your work with a lunch break during which you may return home, or go to your child's daycare center to nurse. Alternatively, your caregiver might bring the child to your work place.

If these situations are not possible to arrange, there are now wonderful and relatively inexpensive pumps (compare them with the price of buying formula) available to the public. Or, you may prefer to rent a pump. In some cases, insurance companies will even cover the cost of a pump rental or purchase because it will save them money in the long run to have healthier babies on their plans.

Using a good quality electric pump it is possible to pump 8–10 ounces of milk in 15 minutes. Battery pumps are also available, and they can be used in a vehicle or in a rest room. It may take longer for newer mothers, and you should plan to pump at least every 4 hours. Beware of cheap low-grade machines, some of which are manufactured by formula companies. They can cause soreness, and probably will not pump sufficient quantities of milk. Remember that pumping is a learned art, and may take time to get perfected. If you do not receive the amount of milk you anticipated, try again, or try a different pump.

If none of these possibilities work for you, you might consider nursing when you are at home and having a caregiver provide a bottle of artificial milk when you are at work. This method should be approached very carefully, however, to avoid depleting the mother's milk supply and endangering the health of the infant.

Myth 14: Night Nursing Causes Dental Problems

Reality: Generally, the worries about babies getting cavities through nighttime milk consumption arise from the practice of leaving babies to sleep with bottles of formula or juice. When this is done harmful bacteria have unlimited access to these sugary mediums and will thrive in the baby's mouth. The acids excreted by the bacteria cause tooth decay. Such decay has been seen occasionally in breastfed babies if these children happen to fall into a small category of people with easily decayed teeth. For most children night nursing will not be a problem.

One advantage that the human nipple provides over an artificial one is that it delivers the milk further toward the back of the mouth, past the teeth. Artificial nipples deliver the milk into the front and middle of the mouth where it can cause decay. Also, the human nipple does not continue to drip milk when it is not being sucked. In contrast, bottles will drip milk all night if left in the bed with the baby. Reminder: no baby should ever be left alone with a propped-up bottle!

If you notice anything strange looking happening to your child's teeth consult a breastfeeding-supportive dentist for help.

Myth 15: Breastfeeding Will Ruin Your Sex Life

Reality: Some people fear that the intimacy that a mother maintains with her child through breastfeeding will displace her needs for intimacy with her partner. This is partially due to our society's viewing of the female breast as a sex organ, rather than a source of nutrition. There is no reason that a breast can't perform both functions. In fact, whether a woman chooses to breastfeed or not, she may find her libido considerably diminished for weeks or months following a birth. It is unrealistic and unfair to expect any new mother who is recovering from a birth; nursing or bottle-feeding around the clock; getting up at night to diaper, rock and soothe the baby; and cooking, cleaning, and chauffeuring to have much interest in sex. If she has an extra half-hour in the evening she will probably choose to use it to sleep! Any tasks that her mate can assist her with will contribute to the deepening of their relationship. If a breastfeeding mother's partner is respectful of the importance of the breastfeeding relationship, and able to assist with things such as diaper changes and nighttime parenting duties, the new mother's sexuality will gradually resurface.

Myth 16: You Have to Have a Good Diet or Your Milk Won't Nourish the Baby Properly

Reality: Surprisingly, new studies have shown this to be untrue. Even women who are getting poor nutrition can usually produce adequate quality milk. However, they may not be able to produce as much of milk as women who are eating well. Needless to say, it's best to eat right during pregnancy and while you're breastfeeding. Occasional lapses, however, are nothing to worry about.

Myth17: Breastfeeding Makes You Fat

Reality: Breastfeeding will certainly not prevent you from getting back to your pre-pregnancy weight. In fact, breastfeeding uses an extra 300 to 500 calories every day. It's up to the mother how many of those calories she chooses to obtain through eating additional food or through burning off her available body fat. It is wise to lose weight gained during pregnancy gradually whether or not you choose to breastfeed. It may take some women longer than others, and it is important to remember that your body has been through a lot, and is still working hard to provide nourishment for your baby. You should not be losing more than a half a pound to a pound per week or you may affect your milk supply. This is a time to be kind to yourself!

Myth 18: Breastfeeding Deprives Your Mate and Other Friends and Family of Their Chance to Bond with the Baby

Reality: There are lots of ways to bond with a new born. Soothing, rocking, diapering, and burping the new baby are only a few of these activities. Anyone can participate in them without depriving the child of it's optimal nutrition and nurturing.

Myth 19: Breastfed Newborns Need Vitamin and Mineral Supplements

Reality: Not true. No vitamin or mineral supplements should be given to breastfed babies until at least six months. New studies are currently being conducted as to whether or not such supplements should be given after six months. Historically, before such supplements were invented, many breastfed babies survived and thrived for the duration of breastfeeding, which could last to three years or older. This is not to say that supplementation is not a good idea after a certain age. It is simply not yet clear what that age is. At least until your baby is 6 months old, you can be assured that your breastmilk will provide for all of her nutritional needs.

Myth 20: You Can't Take Any Medication While You're Breastfeeding

Reality: While there are a few medications that should absolutely not be used during the breastfeeding portion of a woman's life, most can be taken safely. It is important that your doctor checks actual research rather than simply relying on the standard instructions that are issued with the prescription. Most prescription drugs instructions automatically caution against being taken by pregnant or breastfeeding mothers. This warning is issued to prevent liability, and is often overly cautious. It's also a good idea to ask your doctor about non-prescription drugs. Some of them are not appropriate for nursing or pregnant women.

Myth 21: Breastfeeding Ties You Down

Reality: It is true that breastfed babies are dependent upon their mothers for their nutrition. This does not mean that a breastfeeding mother must remain house bound and attached to her baby twenty-four hours a day. After you have recovered from the birth, it is not only possible but usually a lot of fun to take your baby with you on errands, visits to friends, walks in the park, and other outings. Now that it has been clearly established that women have a right to breastfeed in all public spaces, and with the advent of excellent breast pumps, the possibilities for nursing mothers to fully participate in activities outside the home are almost unlimited. It is also nice not to have the added burden of caring around all that formula paraphernalia. If you choose to express some of your milk ahead of time you can easily spend time apart from your baby without relying on artificial substitutes.

Obviously, taking your baby with you on outings will probably mean you'll be nursing him or her in front of others, and maybe in public. Some women feel funny about nursing in front of strangers, or even friends and family members, probably because the sight of a nursing mother is not something they themselves are used to seeing.

As countless mothers will attest, however, it's rare that anyone will stare or say something to you while you're breastfeeding; more likely they'll just look the other way, or not even notice that you're nursing! Breastfeeding in public can be very discreet, especially if you wear clothes that are specially designed for nursing mothers. In general, the more natural your attitude the less you'll notice the reaction of others. If you are hesitant about breastfeeding in public, just remember—it's what breasts are made for, and, like so many other things, the more you do it the easier it will be.

Myth 22: After a Year, Breastmilk Loses All of It's Nutritional Value

Reality: This belief is a total myth, as is evidenced by the recently released guidelines of the American Academy of Pediatricians, which recommend breastfeeding for at least one year. While many people are now aware that breastmilk is the perfect, complete source of nutrition for babies under six months of age, not everyone is aware that breastmilk continues to provide perfect nutrition as long as the mother continues to breastfeed. Breastmilk tailors itself to the needs of a child from birth until weaning. There is no need to worry that at some point the milk will become worthless. It will always contain valuable nutrients, hormones, and immunities. It will always be easier to digest than the milk of another species. As you gradually add new foods to your child's diet, you can be assured that your child is getting excellent nutrition, even on those days when she may choose not to eat much solid food at all.

Myth 23: Serious Athletes Can't Breastfeed

Reality: While it may be uncomfortable to run, dance, or perform strenuous physical activity with very full breasts, it is certainly possible to nurse or pump prior to engaging in such activities. Exercise does not "sour" your milk. Immediately following a vigorous exercise session the lactic acid content in you milk may increase and slightly alter the taste of your milk. However, within an hour or two the lactic acid passes out of the milk again, leaving it tasting just fine. Also, some researches suggest showering off after a workout to get rid of salty tasting sweat. And remember, it's wise to start back to a previously established exercise regimen gradually, whether breastfeeding or not.

Myth 24: Adoptive Mothers Can't Breastfeed

Reality: As surprising as this may seem, you do not have to give birth to a child to produce milk. Many adoptive mothers have successfully developed their ability to produce milk through pumping, putting the baby to their breast and allowing it to suckle, and use of a supplementary feeding system designed to give the baby artificial milk until the mother can begin to produce her own. In some cases only a little milk will be obtained. In others, the majority of the baby's nutrition can be provided from the adoptive mother's body.

Myth 25: You Can't Breastfeed after Menopause

Reality: Interestingly, women can continue to produce milk after they are no longer fertile, and have been known to do so into their eighties! There is no change in the quality of the milk, and many wet nurses have continued to practice their profession well past menopause.

Myth 26: Breastfeeding Clothes and Pumps End Up Costing as Much as Formula

Reality: First of all, you don't need any special clothes or paraphernalia to breastfeed successfully. Yes, if you plan to pump you should buy or rent a good, reputable model. Yes, you'll need storage bags and bottles, although you'd need even more to formula feed. Yes, it's nice to have a few specially designed nursing tops, bras and a nursing pillow. Reusable nursing pads are also helpful, and disposable nursing pads are nice the first few weeks.

However, even with these items taken into consideration, they do not come close to the expense of formula. Plus, there are all the added medical expenses you may have to deal with if you formula feed. Also, when you breastfeed you can reuse most of the items you purchase for one child with the next. With formula, it's just as expensive every time.

It is also possible to purchase sewing patterns and make your own nursing clothes and baby sling if you want to, or create your own pads out of cotton diapers. A T-shirt with a convenient slit cut in the middle can provide extra coverage under any pull-up or button down blouse. Nursing bras are great, but for many women a front closing cotton bra works just as well. Use your imagination!

Compare the costs of breastfeeding and formula feeding in Table 4.1.

The difference between breastfeeding and formula feeding adds up to $2,283. And remember, you can use those nursing clothes again, then consign them or pass them on to a friend. With formula, it's just as expensive with every child.

These figures don't take into account possible future orthodontic problems, or other more serious adult disease issues associated with bottle feeding. Of course, the real bottom line is that no price can be put on the special intimacy that exists between a nursing mother and child!

Table 4.1. Cost Comparisons of Breastfeeding and Formula Feeding.

No-Frills Style Breastfeeding	Optional Breast-feeding Expenses	Approximate Costs of Formula Feeding
No pump	Pump: $40–200	Formula: $1,200 (Approximate average)
No special clothes	Bras (2): $60 Pads (reusable): $12 Tops (2): $50 Dress (1): $60	Added medical expenses: $1,500 (based on Aetna employee research results)
No equipment	Nursing pillow: $35	
Total cost: $0.00	Total: $257–417 (A one-time expense)	Total: $2,700 (For just one year)

Chapter 5

Are Breastfed Babies Smarter?

In the debate over whether babies should be on the breast or bottle, few points may prove as persuasive as the results of a new study indicating that breastfeeding is associated with detectable increases in child cognitive ability and educational achievement.

The study was reported in the January 1998 issue of the journal *Pediatrics* that is published by the American Academy of Pediatrics. The report is by L. John Horwood and David M. Fergusson from the Christchurch School of Medicine in Christchurch, New Zealand.

The study looked at the relationships between the duration of breastfeeding—how long children were on the breast—and their cognitive ability and academic achievement over a period of 8–18 years. The data were collected in the course of an eighteen–year longitudinal study beginning at birth of over 1000 children.

From birth to one year of age, information was collected on maternal breastfeeding practices. Then, over the years the children were tested on a range of measures of cognitive and academic performance. These included "measures of child intelligence quotient; teacher ratings of school performance; standardized tests of reading comprehension, mathematics, and scholastic ability; pass rates in school leaving examinations; and leaving school without qualifications."

Longer breastfeeding was found to be associated with consistent and statistically significant increases in:

"Do Breastfed Babies Do Better? Is Cognitive Ability and Academic Achievement Enhanced?" ©1998, reprinted with permission of MedicineNet, Inc. www.medicinenet.com.

- Intelligence quotient of the children (tested at age 8–9 years.)

- Reading comprehension (tested at age 10–13 years.)

- Mathematical ability (tested at age 10–13 years.)

- Scholastic ability (tested at age10–13 years.)

- Teacher ratings of reading and mathematics (at 8–12 years.)

- Higher levels of attainment in school final examinations.

There were differences between the mothers who breastfed and those who bottle-fed. The mothers who chose to breastfeed as a group tended to be older, to be better educated, and to be from upper socio-economic status families. They tended to be in a two-parent family, did not smoke during pregnancy, and enjoyed above average income and living standards. The rates of breastfeeding also increased with increasing birth weight.

To take these various factors into account, statistical regression adjustments were made for maternal and other factors associated with breastfeeding. Nonetheless, the duration of breastfeeding remained a significant predictor of later cognitive or educational outcomes.

Breastfeeding, it is concluded, is associated with small but detectable increases in the cognitive ability and educational achievement children. These effects are reflected in a range of measures including standardized tests, teacher ratings, and academic outcomes in high school. The beneficial effects of breastfeeding in the New Zealand study were long lived and extended throughout childhood into young adulthood.

The New Zealand study is not alone in suggesting that breastfeeding helps children's cognitive abilities and academic achievement. Longitudinal studies have consistently shown that breastfed babies do better in these respects than bottle-fed babies.

What makes the difference? Is it the experience of being on the breast? Or is it the breastmilk itself? Data from an experimental study of pre-term (premature) babies show that children whose mothers elect to express their own breastmilk later have higher developmental scores and higher intelligence quotients. Thus, the breastmilk itself appears beneficial.

What is in breastmilk that is so good for the brain? Research has suggested that the helpful factors may be long-chain polyunsaturated fatty acids including, in particular, docosahexaenoic acid (DHA). When DHA was added to infant formulas, pre-term babies appeared to show better visual acuity and cognitive abilities.

The New Zealand investigators observe that their findings "underwrite the need to encourage breastfeeding and/or to continue to develop improved infant formulas with properties more similar to those of human milk...." They do believe that their results most likely "reflect the effects of polyunsaturated fatty acid levels and, particularly, DHA levels on early development."

The Nutrition Information Center of New York Hospital-Cornell Medical Center and Memorial Sloan-Kettering Cancer Center recently advised that DHA is "included in infant formulas worldwide, but not in the US" (underlined in the advisory). Assuming DHA is required for optimal brain development—a reasonable conclusion at this time—the question arises. Why are infant formulas in the United States not supplemented with DHA?

Chapter 6

Breastfeeding:
A Matter of Survival?

Infant Health

Breastfeeding saves up to six million lives every year. Optimal breastfeeding (exclusive breastfeeding for the first six months of life and continued breastfeeding with appropriate complementary foods through at least the second year of life) could save an additional one to two million infants. Why?

Immunities

Breastfeeding is the infant's first "immunization" against infectious diseases. Exclusively breastfed infants have 2.5 times fewer episodes of childhood diseases. Infants who are not breastfed are up to twenty-five times more likely to die from diarrhea and nearly three times more likely to die from acute respiratory infections than those who are exclusively breastfed.

Nutrition

Breastfeeding alone is the best nutrition for the first six months of life, and remains an excellent staple food for up to two years or more. Breastmilk changes composition to meet the child's nutritional growth needs and contains a host of specialized nutritional and immunological properties that enhance child growth and development.

"Breastfeeding and Child Survival," an undated publication of the United States Agency for International Development (USAID), www.usaid.gov.

35

Child Spacing

Breastfeeding contributes to child spacing, which is associated with decreased child mortality. Women who breastfeed have longer natural child spacing.

Future Health

Breastfeeding protects beyond the early months of life. Breastfeeding decreases the incidence of childhood cancer and diabetes while improving the child's psychological development and intelligence.

Maternal Health

Breastfeeding contributes to safe motherhood by helping to reduce postpartum bleeding and also decreases the risk of breast and ovarian cancer and brittle bones when the mother is older.

Breastfeeding increases child spacing in developing countries by reducing a woman's total postpartum fertility as much as the use of all modern contraceptive methods combined. The Lactational Amenorrhea Method or LAM (defined as no return of menses, and full breastfeeding up to six months postpartum), provides about 98% protection against pregnancy.

Breastfeeding empowers women and enables them to feel confident as caretakers and promotes their ability to exercise preventive health care practices.

Community Development

Breastfeeding benefits the community as well because it:

- Contributes to economic development by decreasing the amount of foreign exchange spent on breastmilk substitutes and bottles, and reduces health care costs associated with bottle-fed infants.

- Protects the environment. When babies are not breastfed, scarce resources such as water and fuel are wasted on bottle-feeding and can increase pollution.

- Saves scarce financial resources and is food security. Without the estimated twenty million metric tons of breastmilk produced annually by women in the developing world (over 10% of the fluid milk consumed worldwide) infant feeding costs would be $15 billion each year. Breastfeeding provides total food security for infants up to six months of age.

Why Support Breastfeeding Now?

There is a worldwide decline in optimal breastfeeding. Very few mothers practice optimal breastfeeding for the infant's first six months of life (i.e., no teas, water, sugar water, or other foods or liquids are given to the infant). In Kenya, almost 90% of mothers exclusively breastfeed their infants at birth, but after one month only 25% of the mothers exclusively breastfeed. In Latin America, the percentage of mothers who initiate exclusive breastfeeding ranges from 84% (Mexico) to 98% (Bolivia), but exclusive breastfeeding until six months ranges from only about 1% (Brazil) to a peak of about 10% (Bolivia).

The lack of optimal breastfeeding practices contributes to increased infant and under five child morbidity and mortality, reduced world food supply, and increased population growth. Many factors influence a woman's ability to breastfeed and often prevent families from making informed choices:

- fewer traditional support systems for breastfeeding,

- employment policies that do not support breastfeeding,

- shifts in societal norms,

- increased inappropriate baby formula marketing,

- inappropriate feeding practices, and

- a lack of trained health personnel to promote breastfeeding.

Global Efforts

International organizations are renewing their interest in breastfeeding, since numerous studies have confirmed that breastfeeding saves lives. International consensus on the importance of breastfeeding and on optimal breastfeeding was reached at several noteworthy meetings over the past two decades, including the World Health Organization Conference in 1981, when the Code for Marketing of Breastmilk Substitutes was determined; the 1990 United Nations World Summit for Children; and the Innocenti Conference and Declaration.

Part Two

Preparing to Breastfeed

Chapter 7

Who Breastfeeds?

Breastfeeding Practices among American Women

Breastfeeding Rates Past and Present

Breastfeeding is generally accepted as the ideal form of infant nutrition, and major medical associations and governmental agencies have taken strong positions promoting it. Despite this, breastfeeding rates are barely higher today than they were fifteen years ago.

At the turn of the century, more than 90% of American mothers breastfed their children, but breastfeeding rates declined to a low of 25% in the late 1960s. With a new understanding of the health benefits came a resurgence of breastfeeding, peaking at 60% in the early 1980s. Rates gradually declined to just above 50% in the early 1990s, bouncing back slightly to 62% in 1997.

Unfortunately, this 62% represents only the mothers who are breastfeeding at hospital discharge, both exclusively (no added formula) and partially (with added formula). In 1997, a larger proportion of breastfeeding mothers were already mixing breast and bottle

Information for this chapter was excerpted from the following documents. "If Breastfeeding Is So Wonderful, Why Aren't More Women Doing It?" by Alicia Dermer, M.D., I.B.C.L.C. ©1998–2000 by Joel R. Cooper, http://medicalreporter. health.org; reprinted with permission. "Blueprint for Action on Breastfeeding," U.S. Department of Health and Human Services 2000, www.4woman.gov. "WIC Infant Feeding Practices Study: Breastfeeding Duration, Attitudes and Practices," U.S. Department of Agriculture's Women, Infants, and Children Program, November 1997.

at hospital discharge. In 1998, 64% of all mothers breastfed in the early postpartum period and only 29% breastfed at six months postpartum.

Despite the American Academy of Pediatrics (AAP) recommendations that breastmilk should be the sole source of infant nutrition for about the first six months, only a third of mothers who initiate breastfeeding continue to do so for six months, and even fewer breastfeed that long exclusively. Currently, about 80% of American babies are fully formula-fed at six months, and about half of six-month-old breastfed babies also receive formula. Only about 10% of American babies are exclusively breastfed at six months according to the AAP recommendations.

Ethnic, Socioeconomic, and Regional Differences in Breastfeeding Rates

Racial and ethnic disparities in breastfeeding are wide despite substantial increases in breastfeeding rates in the last decade. More white mothers breastfeed than their minority counterparts, and younger less educated women are more likely to bottle feed. It is possible that the increased asthma and diabetes among African Americans is to some extent due to the low rates of breastfeeding, especially among inner city dwellers. In 1998, 45% of African American mothers breastfed their infants in the early postpartum period; 66% of Hispanic mothers and 68% of white mothers did so. No group of women reached the goal of breastfeeding for five to six months postpartum (50%), and again, disparities exist across racial and ethnic groups. (See Table 7.1).

Breastfeeding Practices among Women Participating in the Women, Infants, and Children Program (WIC)

Breastfeeding Rates among WIC Women Mothers Vary

Thirty-one percent of WIC mothers initiated breastfeeding. One-half of breastfeeding WIC mothers stop breastfeeding by the end of the second month, and only 16 percent of all WIC mothers continue breastfeeding until their infant is five months old.

Among the WIC mothers who initiate breastfeeding, some subgroups breastfeed for longer durations than others.

- African American and white mothers are less likely than others to breastfeed until their infant is five months old.

- Mothers who are young and who have low levels of education are likely to stop breastfeeding earlier than other mothers. For example, one-half of breastfeeding mothers who are not yet twenty years old stop breastfeeding by nineteen days after the birth.

- Mothers who were born outside the United States breastfeed longer than other mothers. For example, one-half of the breastfeeding WIC mothers who were born abroad continue breastfeeding ninety-six days or longer after the birth of the infant.

- Mothers who have more than a high school education breastfeed longer than other mothers.

Table 7.1. Racial and Ethnic Disparities in Breastfeeding Rates and Healthy People 2010 Breastfeeding Objectives for the Nation

Time Period	1998 Baseline Percent (%)	2010 Target
In early postpartum period		
All women	64	75
Black or African American	45	75
Hispanic or Latino	66	75
White	68	75
At six months		
All women	29	50
Black or African American	19	50
Hispanic or Latino	28	50
White	31	50
At one year		
All women	16	25
Black or African American	9	25
Hispanic or Latino	19	25
White	17	25

Large Proportions of WIC Infants Who Are Breastfed Also Receive Formula

Formula supplementation of breastfeeding WIC infants starts very early in life. One-fourth of breastfeeding WIC infants are given formula during the first five days of life and one-half are given formula during the first sixteen days of life. At any given month during the first year of life, only about one-half or fewer of breastfeeding WIC mothers breastfeed without supplementing with formula. At one month of age, only 13 percent of all WIC infants are breastfed without formula, another 20 percent are fed breastmilk and formula, and almost two-thirds are fed formula only.

Some subgroups of WIC mothers are more likely than other subgroups to supplement breastmilk with formula. For example, African American mothers and young mothers are more likely to supplement breastmilk with formula. One-half of African American mothers who breastfeed supplement their breastmilk with formula by the time their infants are twelve days old. Breastfeeding mothers who have others care for their infants are more than twice as likely to give formula to their infants than the breastfeeding mothers who care for their infants themselves.

Breastfeeding WIC Mothers Who Supplement with Formula Are Almost 2.5 Times More Likely to Stop Breastfeeding

The difference in breastfeeding duration between the mothers who supplement with formula and those who do not supplement is large. WIC mothers who do not supplement breastmilk with formula are more likely to breastfeed their infants for longer durations than those who do supplement their breastmilk with formula. Almost one-half of the mothers who do not supplement breastmilk with formula are predicted to continue breastfeeding for five months, compared with only 16 percent of the mothers who supplement with formula.

Mothers who believe that breastfeeding is beneficial are less likely to supplement breastfeeding with formula and are also less likely to stop breastfeeding than the mothers who do not believe that breastfeeding is beneficial.

Breastfeeding Mothers Differ from Non-Breastfeeding Mothers in Their Attitudes and Beliefs about Breastfeeding

Non-breastfeeding mothers are significantly less likely to express positive attitudes towards most issues concerning breastfeeding, and are generally more likely to say that they are "not sure" about various statements abut consequences of breastfeeding. Attitudes and beliefs about breastfeeding also vary considerably by race and ethnicity. African American mothers report the most concern about barriers to breastfeeding, and Hispanic mothers report the most awareness of the benefits of breastfeeding.

Attitudes and beliefs about breastfeeding are linked to breastfeeding practices and breastfeeding duration. Mothers who report more positive attitudes towards breastfeeding are less likely to supplement breastfeeding with formula and less likely to stop breastfeeding. In fact, the differences in breastfeeding duration of white, African American, and Hispanic mothers are almost entirely due to the reported differences in beliefs and attitudes towards breastfeeding.

Beliefs about Milk Supply Affect Mother's Duration of Breastfeeding

Mothers who believe that they do not have sufficient milk, or that there is something wrong with their milk, are more likely to supplement breastfeeding with formula and are more likely to stop breastfeeding than mothers who do not report such problems with their milk.

The percentages of breastfeeding mothers who report nursing problems decrease over time. In the first month, 34 percent of the mothers think that they do not have enough milk and 10 percent think that something is wrong with the milk. During the first month following the birth, thinking that one does not have enough breastmilk is the second most common nursing problem reported by the WIC mothers, following sore nipples.

Chapter 8

Frequently Asked Questions about Breastfeeding

Why should I breastfeed?

More than two decades of research have established that breastmilk is the best or most complete form of nutrition for infants and that it protects infants from a wide array of infectious and non-infectious diseases. Some of these include diarrhea, respiratory tract infection, otitis media or ear infection, pneumonia, urinary infection, necrotizing enterocolitis (damage to the intestine and colon), and invasive bacterial infection. Breastfed infants, compared with formula-fed infants, also seem to have stronger immune systems to fight infection. This results in lower rates of chronic childhood diseases such as diabetes, celiac disease, inflammatory bowel disease, childhood cancer, and allergies and asthma. As a result, breastfed babies have lower rates of hospital admissions. Some studies also suggest that the type of fatty acids available in breastmilk enhances brain growth and development in infants, giving them earlier visual acuity and cognitive function.

How is breastmilk different from formula?

Breastmilk has greater nutritional value than infant formula. Human milk contains just the right amount of fat, sugar, water, and

Published 2001 by the Office on Women's Health, Department of Health and Human Services. The information was adapted from "Breastfeeding Best Bet for Babies" by Rebecca D. Williams, *FDA Consumer* October 1995, and from the Department of Health and Human Services' Office on Women's Health's 2000 "Blueprint for Action on Breastfeeding."

protein for human digestion, brain development, and growth. Cow's milk contains a different type of protein that may be good for calves, but human infants can have difficulty digesting it. Bottle-fed infants tend to be fatter than are breastfed infants, but not necessarily healthier.

Breastmilk also contains immunologic agents or the mother's antibodies to disease. These antibodies are transferred to the infant and act against bacteria, viruses, and parasites. Anti-inflammatory agents in breastmilk help to regulate the body's immune system response against infection. Also, a breastfed baby's digestive tract contains large amounts of *Lactobacillus bifidus*, beneficial bacteria that prevent the growth of harmful organisms. Since the infant's immune system is not fully mature until about two years of age, breastmilk provides an advantage that formula-fed infants do not have.

Human milk straight from the breast is always sterile, and is never contaminated by polluted water or dirty bottles, which can lead to diarrhea in the infant.

For how long should you breastfeed your baby?

The Surgeon General, in the newly released Blueprint for Action on Breastfeeding, recommend that babies be breastfed exclusively for the first four to six months of life, preferably six months, and ideally through the first year of life. Protection against infection is strongest during the first several months of life for infants who are breastfed exclusively. Breastfeeding into the second six months of life protects against infection, and longer duration of breastfeeding may provide an even stronger protective effect.

The only acceptable alternative to breastmilk is infant formula. The guidelines from the American Academy of Pediatrics state that solid foods can be introduced when the baby is four to six months old, to complement the breastmilk diet. In the first six months, water, juice, and other foods are generally unnecessary for breastfed infants. A baby should drink breastmilk or formula—not cow's milk—for a full year.

Can a baby be allergic to her mother's milk?

Human milk contains at least 100 ingredients not found in formula. Healthy babies are not allergic to their mother's milk, although they may have a reaction to something the mother eats. If she eliminates it from her diet, the problem usually resolves itself.

Does the baby know the difference between breastmilk and formula?

Many psychologists believe the nursing baby enjoys a sense of security from the warmth and presence of the mother, especially when there's skin-to-skin contact during feeding. Parents of bottle-fed babies may be tempted to prop bottles in the baby's mouth, with no human contact during feeding. But a nursing mother must cuddle her infant closely many times during the day. Nursing becomes more than a way to feed a baby, it's a source of warmth and comfort.

Why is breastfeeding good for mothers?

Breastfeeding is good for new mothers as well as for their babies. There are no bottles to sterilize and no formula to buy, measure, and mix. It may be easier for a nursing mother to lose the pounds of pregnancy as well, since nursing uses up extra calories. Lactation (breastfeeding) also stimulates the uterus to contract back to its original size and reduces postpartum bleeding. Breastfeeding also may lower the risk of pre-menopausal breast cancer and ovarian cancer.

A nursing mother must get needed rest, otherwise her body may decrease milk production. She must sit down, put her feet up, and relax every few hours to nurse. Nursing at night is easy. No one has to stumble to the refrigerator for a bottle and warm it while the baby cries. If she's lying down, a mother can doze while she nurses.

Nursing also is nature's contraceptive—although not a very reliable one. Frequent nursing suppresses ovulation, making it less likely for a nursing mother to ovulate, menstruate, or get pregnant. There are no guarantees, however. Mothers who don't want more children right away should use contraception even while nursing. Hormone injections and implants are safe during nursing, as are all barrier methods of birth control. The labeling on birth control pills says that until the baby is weaned, another form of contraception should be used if possible. Estrogen may be harmful to infants. The only safe oral contraceptive for nursing mothers is a progestin-only birth control pill, also called the "mini-pill." Unlike oral contraceptives that contain both estrogen and progesterone, the mini-pill only contains progesterone and will not affect milk production.

Breastfeeding also is economical. Even though a nursing mother works up a big appetite and consumes extra calories, the extra food for her is less expensive than buying formula for the baby. Nursing saves money while providing the best nourishment possible.

49

Who else benefits from breastfeeding?

Breastfeeding is not only good for infants and mothers, but can benefit the family, the health care system, the employer, and the nation as a whole. Even after accounting for the costs of breast pump equipment, if necessary, families can save several hundreds of dollars they would have spent on formula. Because breastfed infants are sick less often, they require fewer visits to the doctor, prescriptions, and hospitalizations. This results in lower medical costs for the nation. In companies with established lactation programs, absenteeism rates and medical costs are lower, and productivity is higher.

Is there any time when a woman shouldn't breastfeed?

Most common illnesses, such as colds, flu, skin infections, or diarrhea, cannot be passed through breastmilk. In fact, if a mother has an illness, her breastmilk will contain antibodies to it that will help protect her baby from those same illnesses.

A few viruses can pass through breastmilk, however. HIV, the virus that causes AIDS, is one of them. Women who are HIV positive should not breastfeed. Also, women with human T-cell leukemia virus type 1 (HTLV-1) should not breastfeed because of the risk of transmission to the child. Hepatitis C is another virus that may be transmitted through breastfeeding if the mother has cracked or bleeding nipples. Otherwise, the risk of Hepatitis C is the same whether breastfed or bottle-fed.

An infant born with a condition called galactosemia cannot metabolize lactose, a sugar found in all mammalian milk, and must be fed plant-derived formula. Infants with phenylketonuria can be successfully breastfed, but doing so requires special clinical management.

Can breast cancer be passed through nursing?

Breast cancer is not passed through breastmilk. Women who have had breast cancer can usually breastfeed from the unaffected breast. There is some concern that the hormones produced during pregnancy and lactation may trigger a recurrence of cancer, but so far this has not been proven. Studies have shown, however, that breastfeeding a child reduces a woman's chance of developing breast cancer later.

Do breast implants affect breastfeeding?

It is not known whether breastfeeding by women who have breast implants has an effect on the nursing infant. Many women with implants lactate successfully. Women who have had reduction mammoplasty may not be able to lactate if the glandular tissue has been removed or the connection between it and the nipple is interrupted.

What are some of the challenges of breastfeeding?

For all its health benefits, breastfeeding can be challenging. In the early weeks, it can be painful if it is not done properly. A woman's nipples may become sore or cracked if she allows her infant to latch on to the nipple instead of the areola. She may experience engorgement more than a bottle-feeding mother, when the breasts become so full of milk that they're hard and painful. She can reduce the risk of painful engorgement by using proper latch-on and positioning, as well as by allowing the baby to nurse on demand. Engorgement can be relieved by frequent feedings, massaging the breast, and by applying warm or cold compresses between feedings. Nursing women may also develop clogged milk ducts, which can lead to mastitis, a painful infection of the breast. While most nursing problems can be solved with home remedies, mastitis requires prompt medical care.

How can someone go back to working outside the home and still breastfeed?

Women who plan to go back to work soon after birth will have to plan carefully if they want to breastfeed. If her job allows, a new mother can pump her breastmilk several times during the day and refrigerate or freeze it for the baby to take in a bottle later. Or, some women alternate nursing at night and on weekends with daytime bottles of formula. Her milk production can adapt to the alternating schedule.

If a woman's workplace does not have a lactation program, she should ask her supervisor or Human Resources Department to arrange for her needs. Working mothers who are breastfeeding need a private, clean, relaxing environment where they:

- can pump milk,
- have an adequate storage place for the milk,
- have adequate breaks during the day to pump,
- have more flexible work schedules, and, ideally,
- have onsite child care facilities.

If an employer gives a woman resistance to her needs, she can refer the employer to the Surgeon General's Blueprint for Action on Breastfeeding, which encourages employers to make accommodations for breastfeeding mothers.

Is it safe to take medications while breastfeeding?

Most medications have not been tested in nursing women, so no one knows exactly how a given drug will affect a breastfed child. Since very few problems have been reported, however, most over-the-counter and prescription drugs—taken in moderation and only when necessary—are considered safe.

Even mothers who must take daily medication for conditions such as epilepsy, diabetes, or high blood pressure can usually breastfeed. They should first check with the child's pediatrician. To minimize the baby's exposure, the mother can take the drug just after nursing or before the child sleeps.

If I choose to breastfeed, is there any right way to do so?

According to the FDA, the following advice should help make breastfeeding a pleasant experience for the mother and baby.

Get an Early Start

Nursing should begin within an hour after delivery if possible, when an infant is awake and the sucking instinct is strong. Even though the mother won't be producing milk yet, her breasts contain colostrum, a thick, yellowish fluid that contains antibodies to disease.

Use Proper Positioning

The baby's mouth should be wide open. After placing the nipple in the baby's mouth as far back as possible, make sure his or her lips and gums are around the areola and not only on the nipple. This minimizes soreness for the mother. A nurse, midwife, or other knowledgeable person can help her find a comfortable nursing position.

Nurse on demand

Newborns need to nurse frequently, whenever they show signs of hunger, at least every two hours, and not on any strict schedule. Signs of hunger include increased alertness or activity, mouthing, or rooting.

Crying is a late indicator of hunger. Newborns should be nursed approximately eight to twelve times every twenty-four hours until satiety (usually ten to fifteen minutes on each breast.) In the early weeks after birth, non-demanding babies should be aroused to feed if four hours have elapsed since the last nursing. This will stimulate the mother's breasts to produce plenty of milk. Later, the baby can settle into a more predictable routine. But because breastmilk is more easily digested than formula, breastfed babies often eat more frequently than bottle-fed babies.

No Supplements

Nursing babies don't need sugar water or formula supplements. These may interfere with their appetite for nursing, which can lead to a diminished milk supply. The more the baby nurses, the more milk the mother will produce.

Delay Artificial Nipples

A newborn has to learn how to breastfeed. It is best to allow time to establish a good sucking pattern before introducing a pacifier. Artificial nipples require a different sucking action than real ones. Sucking at a bottle could also confuse some babies in the early days.

Air Dry

In the early postpartum period or until her nipples toughen, the mother should air them dry after each nursing to prevent them from cracking, which can lead to infection. If her nipples do crack, the mother can coat them with breastmilk or other natural moisturizers to help them heal. Vitamin E oil and lanolin are commonly used, although some babies may have allergic reactions to them. Proper positioning at the breast can help prevent sore nipples. If the mother is very sore, the baby may not have the nipple far enough back in his or her mouth.

Watch for Infection

Symptoms of breast infection include fever, irritation, and painful lumps and redness in the breast. These require immediate medical attention.

Expect Engorgement

A new mother usually produces lots of milk, making her breasts big, hard, and painful for a few days. To relieve this engorgement, she should feed the baby frequently and on demand until her body adjusts and produces only what the baby needs. In the meantime, the mother can apply warm, wet compresses to her breasts and take warm baths to relieve the pain. She can also express some milk before breastfeeding, either manually or with a breast pump. For severe engorgement, warmth may not help. In this case, she may want to use cold compresses as she expresses milk. Ice packs used between feedings can relieve discomfort and reduce swelling. Pain from engorgement also may be relieved by feeding the baby in more than one position, or gently massaging the breasts from under the arm and down toward the nipple. This will help reduce soreness and ease milk flow. Do not take any medications without approval from your doctor. Acetaminophen (Tylenol) may relieve pain and is safe to take occasionally during breastfeeding.

Eat Right, Get Rest

To produce plenty of good milk, the nursing mother needs a balanced diet that includes five hundred extra calories a day and six to eight glasses of fluid. She should also rest as much as possible to prevent breast infections, which are aggravated by fatigue.

How do I know that my baby is getting enough milk from breastfeeding?

Babies vary in their eating and diaper habits, but the American Academy of Pediatrics advises breastfeeding mothers to watch for certain signs that their babies are getting enough milk. These signs are as follows:

- At least six wet diapers per day and two to five loose yellow stools per day, depending on baby's age. Stools should be loose and have a yellowish color to them. Be sure stools are not white or clay-colored.

- Steady weight gain after the first week of age.

- Pale yellow urine, not deep yellow or orange.

- Sleeping well, yet baby looks alert and healthy when awake.

Where can I find more information?

You can find out more about breastfeeding by contacting any of the organizations listed in Chapter 64, Breastfeeding Resources.

Chapter 9

Breastfeeding Basics

Making Breastmilk

Colostrum is a special milk for the baby's early feedings. It is made by the milk glands starting early in pregnancy. It is thicker than other milk and just what your baby needs for the first few days. Colostrum is the perfect first food for your baby.

During the first 3–4 days your breasts will begin to feel fuller before feedings. The milk glands are changing from making colostrum to making milk. People say the milk is "coming in." The breasts are making MORE milk, because your baby is ready for more.

As the milk comes in, your breasts may become engorged (swollen). Most mothers feel heavier or fuller before feedings but do not get engorged. Breastfeeding at least every 2–3 hours during the day and at least once at night will help keep your breasts comfortable as your milk comes in.

When your baby is about two weeks old (or before), your breasts will get a little softer and smaller. This does NOT mean you have less milk. Your breasts are getting used to holding milk and are less swollen.

Let-Down

As your baby starts to nurse, your milk starts to flow. Several times during a feeding your milk glands release more milk. This is called

An undated publication from North Carolina Department of Health and Human Services Nutri-NET Child Nutrition Information (http://wch.dhhs.state.nc.us). Reprinted with permission.

let-down (or milk ejection reflex). The same hormone that causes the let-down makes your uterus contract (tighten). As your milk lets down, you may also feel your uterus cramp and have heavier vaginal bleeding. After the first few days, the uterus is smaller and you do not feel that cramping anymore. Some mothers feel a tingling or tightening in their breasts with the let-down at the start of each feeding. Some mothers do not feel the let-down but see their babies start to gulp as the milk comes faster.

Making Enough Milk

When you nurse as long and as often as your baby wants, you are telling your breasts how much milk to make. This is often called supply meets demand. Supply meets demand as long as you breastfeed, even when your baby is bigger. Your body makes as much milk as your baby is taking.

Holding Your Baby for Feedings

There are different ways you can hold your baby when breastfeeding. Choose the position that is most comfortable for you.

Football

If you have a Cesarean section, you will probably want to use the football hold or lie down to nurse at first. That will keep the baby off your stomach. Place a pillow or two at your side to raise the baby to the level of your breast. Put the baby on the pillow with her bottom and legs touching the back of the chair (like an "L").

Hold the baby's shoulders in the palm of your hand supporting the base of the baby's head. Use your other hand under the breast to keep it in the baby's mouth.

Across the Lap

Hold the baby's shoulders in the palm of your hand with your arm supporting the baby's bottom. Bring the baby across your lap. Use your other hand under the breast from the side to keep the nipple in the baby's mouth.

Cradle

Cradle the baby in your arm, his tummy against yours. The baby's head will be resting in the bend of your elbow. The baby's whole body is facing you, tummy-to-tummy. Use your other hand to support the breast.

Lying Down

Lie down on your side and pull the baby close to you so that you are facing each other. Some mothers place a pillow or rolled-up towel against the baby's back to keep the baby in position. A pillow behind your back may make you more comfortable. Help the baby latch on to the breast closest to the bed.

Getting Your Baby Latched on

Have pillows or folded blankets under the baby. The baby's hips need to be almost as high as the baby's head. This will help keep the baby's jaw relaxed to nurse without pinching your nipple. As your baby gets older you may not need this support, but it is very helpful at first.

Hold your baby close to you. The baby's ear, shoulder, and hip should be in a straight line. Do not push the baby's head forward. Pushing the head makes it hard for the baby to swallow.

Hold your breast in one hand with your fingers underneath and thumb on top. Have your hand back from the areola (the dark skin around the nipple). Your hand should not get in the way as the baby latches on. The baby needs to get the nipple far back in the mouth to nurse so milk can flow easily.

Line up the baby's lips with your nipple. Touch the lips with your nipple until the baby's mouth opens wide. The baby is looking for something to suck. This is called rooting. Pull the baby quickly onto the breast. Once the baby starts sucking, you will feel a tug on your nipple. It should not hurt after the first few sucks.

If it hurts, start over. Put your finger in the baby's mouth between the gums and take your nipple out. Make sure the baby's mouth is wide open and the tongue is down before the baby latches on again. It is okay to start over several times.

Signs That Breastfeeding Is Going Well

Breastfeeding is going well for you and your baby when:

- You feel a tug, but it does not hurt when the baby sucks.
- Your baby swallows hard after a few strong sucks.
- Your baby is content at the end of the feeding.

- By four days old, your baby has at least six wet diapers, and two to five yellow bowel movements every twenty-four hours.

- Your baby is gaining weight at each checkup.

These are other signs that you may see:

- Your uterus may tighten during or after feedings the first few days after delivery.

- You may feel sleepy or relaxed when your baby nurses.

- You may notice that your breast softens as your baby nurses.

- Your baby's arms and shoulders will relax during feeding.

Chapter 10

The Process of Milk Production

The Anatomy of Milk Production

Your breast is actually a gland which consists of 15–25 separate, branched segments. These are surrounded by supporting and fat tissue. Milk-producing cells line the small, balloon-like alveoli, which are small chambers of milk clustered at the end of each branch. Milk ducts lead from the alveoli to ever larger ducts which widen to the sinuses (milk stores) just behind the opening of the nipple. (See Figure 10.1.)

The milk is not really sucked out of the breast, rather it is milked out of the sinuses behind the nipple. The pressure of the baby's tongue and bottom lip against the sinuses, together with the inner pressure created by the let-down reflex, actually squirts the milk out. A good milking movement of the baby's mouth is possible only when the baby is positioned well.

The Flow of Milk

When your baby is suckling at your breast, this releases hormones that make your milk flow towards the milk stores behind your nipples.

This chapter includes text from the following documents: "Understanding Breastfeeding Supply and Demand," used with permission of the USDA/ARS Children's Nutrition Research Center at Baylor College of Medicine. Excerpts from "How to Breastfeed during an Emergency" by Dr. Elisabet Helsing, Dr. Aileen Robertson, and Tine Dige Vinther; reprinted with permission of the World Health Organization Regional Office for Europe.

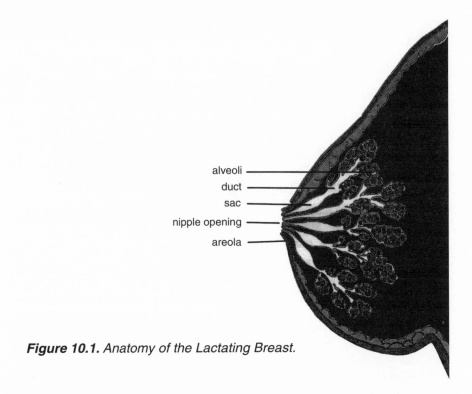

alveoli
duct
sac
nipple opening
areola

Figure 10.1. Anatomy of the Lactating Breast.

This is called the "let-down reflex." The mere sight or thought of your baby may start the reflex and make your milk flow. Conversely, the let-down reflex can be temporarily delayed or inhibited by worry, pain, embarrassment, and other unpleasant feelings. In such cases the milk flow may be interrupted temporarily, from a few minutes to several hours. Remember that this is always temporary and can always be reversed. It is not physically possible to "lose" your milk or your ability to breastfeed.

The more the baby stimulates the breast and hormone release by suckling, the more milk you produce. Also, the more milk is removed from the breast, the more is produced. Conversely, if your baby's suckling is reduced, your milk production also will be reduced. This means that if you try to restrict or regulate breastfeeding to a certain number of feeds or a limited time at the breast, the message you give to your body is to produce a restricted amount, and your baby may not get the milk it actually needs. If instead the baby's appetite and needs are allowed to determine how often and for how long you feed, the milk production will adjust to the baby's need.

Your breast is never completely "empty" of milk. Normally, your baby leaves some milk in the breast. Production goes on very intensely as the baby feeds, and continues after your baby has finished feeding. When the breast is very full of milk, and the alveoli are stretched out like little full balloons, the production of milk slows down.

The composition of your milk changes during a feed, from watery "foremilk" at the beginning to fat, rich "hindmilk" at the end. The composition and amount of milk also change during the day and over the months.

Understanding Breastfeeding Supply and Demand

A nursing baby with an insatiable appetite can cause a first-time mom to doubt more than just her sanity. But, a simple lesson in supply and demand can provide reassurance that her hungry infant is doing exactly as nature intended.

"Sudden increases in infant appetite and feeding frequency should not alarm breastfeeding moms," said Darryl Hadsell, a Ph.D. scientist who studies mammary cell response to lactation-related hormones and nutrient availability at the Children's Nutrition Research Center (CNRC). "Increased demand sets up a biological chain reaction that ensures a mother's milk production keeps pace with her infant's needs for growth and development."

According to Hadsell, the laws of physics require that the concentration of lactose, the milk sugar, remains constant in breastmilk. This means that a mother's body naturally increases milk volume when it steps up production of lactose.

"Lactose production inside milk-producing cells is tied to the synthesis of a key protein that helps turn blood sugar into lactose," Hadsell said. The production of this protein, called alpha-lactalbumin, is under the control of hormones that are released in response to nursing.

Increased feeding frequency causes more of a hormone called prolactin to be released into a mother's bloodstream. This hormone, along with insulin and substances called glucocorticoids, turn on alpha-lactalbumin production, which causes more lactose to be made and leads to greater milk volume.

According to Hadsell, this cascade of events—from demanding infant to hormone-induced increased milk volume—continues until milk supply meets demand. Once it does, then infant hunger, feeding frequency, and family life generally return to normal.

However, a new mom who isn't aware of this natural progression might doubt her body's ability to meet her hungry child's needs and begin supplementing with formula. While this might give temporary relief, it can intensify breastfeeding problems in the long run. "Feeding formula interrupts the nursing cycle and reduces breast emptying, which permits a build up of another protein involved in regulating milk production called the Feedback Inhibitor of Lactation, or FIL," Hadsell said.

A build up of FIL reduces the sensitivity of milk-producing cells to prolactin, which cuts alpha-lactalbumin and lactose production. "In the short run, the effects of FIL on milk volume are reversible if exclusive breastfeeding is soon resumed. But, if the situation becomes chronic, FIL is thought to trigger an actual reduction in the number of breast cells capable of producing milk," he said. "While this is normal during the weaning period, it is not desirable otherwise."

"A new mother can trust her body to respond to her infant's changing nutritional needs if she simply allows her infant to determine the timing and duration of feedings," Hadsell said.

How to Assist the Flow of Milk

- Keep your baby close to your breast and allow it to suckle frequently, even if you believe there is no milk.

- Make sure that your baby is well positioned at your breast.

- Remember that your ability to breastfeed is a strong survival feature, and that the process of making milk is a very simple and robust physiological function.

- Make yourself comfortable before you sit or lie down for a feed.

- If you have problems with the let-down reflex, try if possible to find out which situations you feel stimulate the milk flow and to avoid those that inhibit it.

- Remember that breastfeeding is a good anti-stress therapy for yourself and for the baby.

Chapter 11

Ten Things Expectant Parents Need to Know about Breastfeeding

Breastfeeding Is an Important Health Issue

Hundreds of medical studies have been done on the differing health consequences of breastfeeding and formula feeding. The results are unanimous: every study shows significantly greater instances of illness among artificially-fed babies, even where clean water, adequate supplies of formula, and modern medical care are available. Some of these illnesses are minor and easily curable and some of them are extremely rare regardless of feeding method. Some of them are fairly common and fairly serious (gastroenteritis and pneumonia, among them). And the impact appears to be lifelong: several studies have shown a significant influence on adult illness rates (e.g., both pre- and post-menopausal breast cancer are 25% less common among the population of adult women who were breastfed as infants).

It is not true that all, or even most, formula-fed babies are sick. Nor are all breastfed babies healthy. The studies are epidemiological in nature. When researchers look at different feeding methods among populations and compare disease rates among them, they have consistently found higher disease rates among the population that was fed substitutes for human milk.

It is therefore worth investing some of your time and energy in breastfeeding. Take some steps before your child is born to increase your chances of success. Be prepared to take steps to solve problems that arise. Make a commitment to do whatever you can manage to do to make breastfeeding work for you and your baby. If, despite your best efforts, breastfeeding does not work out, you will at least have the consolation of knowing that you did your best, and that your baby probably got some of the benefits of the earliest feedings.

Breastfeeding Is a Learned Art

If you have grown up around breastfeeding women, you probably know enough to breastfeed without expert help. Indeed, those other breastfeeding women in your life are likely to be the best experts you can turn to for help. However, if you have been raised in a bottle-feeding culture (the U.S. and the U.K. being the most pervasive in their bottle-feeding bias), you may never have even glimpsed another woman breastfeeding.

If you mistakenly think that breastfeeding is simply instinctive, you may not think it necessary to educate yourself about the process and it will be harder for you to accept the help you may need to get started. If, instead, you go into breastfeeding with the knowledge that it must be learned and that you are not trained, you will be able to arm yourself in advance with the knowledge you need to succeed, and you will know when to accept expert help.

Because breastfeeding is a learned art that has been lost to the majority of mothers in a bottle-feeding culture, all mothers should be prepared to deal with some breastfeeding problems. This does not mean obsessing over every horror story that you hear, but it does mean being aware that problems can arise, and learning how to find help if they do.

Find the Best Sources of Information on Breastfeeding

La Leche League International and similar support organizations are the best sources of accurate and helpful information about breastfeeding. If you can afford it, buy a book such as La Leche League's *Breastfeeding: Pure and Simple* that covers all of the basics. You may also be able to find helpful books in your local library or borrow them from a local La Leche League group.

Many Breastfeeding Problems Are Caused by Medical Mismanagement

Ideally, you should be able to choose health care providers that are educated about and supportive of breastfeeding. But that is not always possible. It is an unfortunate fact that, in addition to educating yourself about breastfeeding, you may have to educate your obstetrician, pediatrician, family practice doctor, midwife, maternity floor nurses, and others. You must also be prepared to fend off bad advice and unnecessary procedures that may interfere with breastfeeding.

To avoid misunderstandings, it is advisable to set aside some time in your preparation for childbirth to discuss breastfeeding with your health care providers. Make it plain that you are committed to breastfeeding your baby and that you want to remove all unnecessary barriers to breastfeeding. One of the most important issues to discuss is the avoidance of all artificial nipples in the first days of life. Nipple preference (where a breastfeeding baby learns to prefer an artificial nipple to his mother's) is a leading cause of breastfeeding failure, yet routine bottles and pacifiers are still common in some hospital nurseries. It can't hurt to ask your doctors and hospital to sign a document promising not to use artificial nipples, and make sure that document makes its way into your baby's chart. Then, if supplementary feeds are necessary, they can be administered by cup, spoon, dropper, syringe, or tube.

Some other important issues you might want to discuss with your doctors are:

- What effects will any labor medications have on the initiation of breastfeeding?

- Can cleaning and examination of the baby be postponed until after the baby has had her first feed?

- Can rooming in with the baby be arranged and, if not, will the nursery staff bring the baby to you frequently enough to get breastfeeding started?

- Can circumcision (if such is your choice) be postponed until after breastfeeding has been well established?

- Are there trained lactation consultants on staff at the hospital or pediatrician's office?

- Does a family history of allergies make breastfeeding especially important for the baby?

You might also ask the doctor how she deals with a mother who is concerned about the adequacy of her supply because her baby is nursing every hour. If she responds that formula supplementation is the first line of treatment for this concern, you should not rely upon her advice regarding breastfeeding. Frequent nursing may have nothing to do with inadequate milk supply, and unnecessary supplementation is the fastest road to the end of breastfeeding.

If It Hurts, It Is Likely That Something Is Wrong

Breastfeeding is not supposed to hurt. While some women experience discomfort in the first days of nursing, real pain is almost always a sign that something is wrong. Some possible problems that can cause pain and nipple damage: incorrect latch, incorrect positioning, incorrect sucking, and yeast infection (thrush). These problems can usually be solved, but only if you seek the right kind of help soon enough. If you wait too long, the baby may be hard to retrain, your nipples may be seriously injured, and the joy of breastfeeding may be replaced with dread and misery. And if you seek help from someone who doesn't really know much about breastfeeding, or who doesn't take the time to watch you and your baby nursing, you may be worse off than with no help at all.

The best kind of help is a personal visit with an International Board Certified Lactation Consultant (I.B.C.L.C.). The I.B.C.L.C. is the only internationally-recognized credential showing thorough training and expertise in the diagnosis and treatment of nursing problems. In a personal visit, a lactation consultant can:

- examine your baby and your breasts,
- observe you and your baby nursing to evaluate latch and positioning,
- let your baby suck on her finger to evaluate the baby's sucking behavior,
- listen for the sound of your baby swallowing, and
- talk to you and get a total picture of your nursing relationship.

She can then work with you to put together a treatment plan to solve your breastfeeding problems.

Of course, like any health care professional, a lactation consultant will expect to be paid. If that bothers you, try to remember that the formula to feed a baby for the first year of its life will cost about fifteen times more than a visit with a lactation consultant. Not to mention the risk you run of additional medical expenses that may arise because of the greater risk of illness in formula-fed babies.

Know the Signs of Dehydration

The scariest risk of the early postpartum period with a breastfeeding baby is the risk that the baby's fluid intake will be so low as to cause dehydration. The following are signs of dehydration.

- Fewer than six very wet diapers per day.

- Significant color or odor to the urine (it should be clear and nearly odorless).

- Dry skin that doesn't spring back immediately after being pinched.

- Sunken fontanel (that's the soft spot at the top of the baby's head).

If your baby exhibits any of these symptoms, get immediate medical attention!

If you do have to supplement your baby's fluid intake, remember that cup, spoon, syringe, dropper, and tube feeding are all preferable to a bottle, and expressed breastmilk is preferable to any artificial baby milk.

If the baby is not exhibiting the symptoms of dehydration, has good color, and can be heard swallowing after every couple of sucks, it is unlikely that you are having problems with your supply of milk, regardless of how frequently the baby is nursing. Supplementing with formula at this stage can cause breastfeeding failure. The baby's reduced demand will lead to reduced supply and further supplementation, in a downward spiral toward the complete cessation of breastfeeding.

You Will Need Support to Breastfeed

Support can come in many forms. The most important support for many mothers comes from the baby's father: if he is fully supportive of breastfeeding, it is much easier for the mother to find the strength to breastfeed in a bottle-feeding culture. For some mothers, support can be a relative, friend, or neighbor who has breastfed and who acts as a positive model. For some, it is an organized support group such as La Leche League. For some, it is a lactation consultant or other medical professional who provides expert help when difficulties arise.

Without support, many mothers will quickly abandon any efforts to breastfeed because it makes them feel even more isolated at a time in their lives when the stresses of a new baby have already isolated them.

Your Breasts Are Functional and Their Function Is Feeding Babies

While many of us have grown up believing that our breasts were primarily sexual, the reality is that their sexual function is a cultural construct. The biological reality is that our breasts are for feeding babies. It helps to keep this in mind as you prepare yourself for dealing with people who think there is something indecent about feeding a baby with your breasts. There is absolutely no reason why you should not feed your baby wherever and whenever any bottle-feeding mother would feel comfortable feeding her baby. If the bottle-feeders aren't forced to feed their babies in the bathroom, neither should you.

To avoid unwanted attention, it is wise to learn how to nurse discreetly and to wear clothing that permits easy access to your breasts without disrobing. But try not to let the fact that you take those precautions make you ashamed if someone detects what you are up to. Feeding your baby is not an indecent act no matter where it occurs.

Human Milk Can Be Provided in a Mother's Absence

When mother and baby must be separated, expressing and storing human milk is not only possible but relatively easy. With good hand expression technique or a good quality pump, about fifteen minutes of break time twice a day, and a place to express milk in privacy, most mothers can provide all of their babies' need for milk even if they are working full time. If this is your plan, you will need some additional education and preparation regarding expressing and storing your milk.

It Is Normal to Breastfeed for Two Years or More

Exclusive breastfeeding, in which the baby receives no nourishment other than his or her mother's milk, usually lasts around six months. Somewhere around the second half of the first year, most babies are ready to start eating some other foods. But the transition to a diet that is similar to that of an adult is meant to be gradual, and human milk is a healthy part of a child's diet for some time after the first solids are introduced.

Studies by anthropologists and comparative biologists have revealed that the probable natural weaning age (that is, the age at which no more nursing occurs) of the human species is over 2 ½ years. There is no harm in permitting a child who wants to continue nursing for two years or more to do so. In fact, it is quite common everywhere in the world that bottle feeding is not the cultural norm. The fact that it is not unusual in our culture for a child of three to be drinking milk from a bottle or using a pacifier is a clue that the need to suck is a fundamental human need that does not disappear at six months or one year of age.

Chapter 12

Planning to Breastfeed

There is nothing special you must do while you are pregnant to get ready to breastfeed. You can decide to breastfeed at any time, even after you have your baby. There are some things you can think about and plan for before you begin breastfeeding your baby.

Family and Friends

Sometimes family and friends worry that they will be left out if you breastfeed your baby. They think the baby will love only you. However, babies learn to trust and love the people who come to them when they cry for help. Feeding the baby usually takes about 30 minutes. Everything else can be done by anyone who cares for the baby.

Your family and friends can:

- Pick up the baby when he or she cries.

- Change the baby's diaper.

- Make the baby comfortable in clean, dry clothes.

- Take the baby for a walk.

- Talk or sing soothingly.

- Snuggle with the baby.

An undated publication from North Carolina Department of Health and Human Services Nutri-NET Child Nutrition Information (http://wch.dhhs. state.nc.us). Reprinted with permission.

71

- Rock or swing together.

- Help the baby to burp by gently rubbing or patting his or her back.

- Play peek-a-boo games with the baby.

- Give the baby a warm, relaxing bath.

Someone close to you may be upset, thinking you will undress in public to feed your baby. They do not want to feel embarrassed. Let them know that you can nurse without showing your breast or nurse in private.

You or your family may worry about having enough time for other children when you are breastfeeding. One of the nice things about breastfeeding is that most mothers have a hand free once the baby begins to nurse. You can hug your older child, hold a book to read a story, or even zip a jacket.

Some people may ask you questions about breastfeeding. Remember, they care about you and the baby. You may want to share this book with them.

Nursing around Other People

Not all women feel the same about nursing around other people. You may feel comfortable nursing around other people. Other women may feel embarrassed to breastfeed in front of others. They are afraid that people will see their breasts while nursing. They also worry that nursing will make the people around them feel uncomfortable. All of these feelings are normal.

With some practice, your baby will learn to latch on and nurse easily and you may be comfortable nursing around other people. There are simple ways to cover your breasts while nursing. You can wear oversized tops or unbutton blouses from the waist up. You can put a blanket or a scarf over your shoulder to cover your baby at the breast. You may want to practice breastfeeding in front of a mirror so you can see how you look to others. Some mothers only like to nurse in private. They use a bottle of breast milk or formula when they are around other people.

Going out with Your Baby

Breastfed babies are easy to take with you. You do not need to carry bottles or hurry home when your baby is hungry. Your breastmilk is ready to feed, no matter how long you have been gone.

Young babies nurse about every 2–3 hours. Older babies do not nurse as often. That means your baby will be happy or may sleep for hours between feedings. This is a good time to get a few things done.

Many stores have dressing rooms that are clean and quiet where you can sit and nurse your baby. Churches usually have a cry room, or a quiet classroom where you can nurse. If you are at the clinic and your baby needs to nurse, you can ask for an empty exam room. If you want to nurse privately, nurse your baby in the car. Remember, your baby should always be in a safety seat when the car is moving.

If you do not feel comfortable with any of these ideas, offer a bottle whenever you must feed your baby in public. The bottle can be filled with breastmilk or formula.

Going to Work or School

Many mothers go to work or school and still breastfeed. You can do what works best for you and your baby. Breastfeed when you are at home, and:

- Be away only between feedings, so no milk is needed.

- Pump your breasts once or twice while you are away. Save the milk for the next day's feedings.

- Use formula for the feedings you miss.

Try and nurse your baby as much as you can so that you keep a good milk supply. Ask your sitter not to feed the baby right before you get home so you can breastfeed.

Getting Ready to Breastfeed

Almost every mother can breastfeed her baby. Women who have certain medical problems should not breastfeed. One of these is being HIV positive (having the virus that causes AIDS). Since the HIV virus can go to the baby through breastmilk, the current advice is that HIV positive mothers in the United States should not breastfeed.

Before the baby is born there is nothing special to do to get your nipples ready for breastfeeding. The little bumps around the areola (the darker area around your nipple) make a special oil that keeps your nipples soft and clean. Do not use soap on your nipples. Soap would wash away that oil.

73

Your breasts may get bigger and feel tender. They start making colostrum (early milk) while you are pregnant. Colostrum is a clear, yellow, sticky liquid. Some women leak colostrum while they are pregnant. If your bra sticks to the nipple, wet your bra so it does not hurt when you take it off.

You do not have to wear a bra unless it makes your breasts feel better. If you wear a bra, buy a nursing bra that gives you comfortable support. You may want to see if you can open and close a flap easily with one hand while pretending to hold a baby.

Check Your Nipples

Some nipples stick out when they are touched, and some stay soft or go in. If your nipple goes in when you rub it, you have an inverted nipple. Ask someone at the clinic about getting breast shells to wear inside your bra. The shells may help inverted nipples stick out. They can also be worn between feedings for a few days after the baby is born. Your baby's sucking will bring your nipple out more.

Ask the nurse or nutritionist about breastfeeding classes or groups. When you go to the hospital, tell the nurses that you are going to breastfeed.

Chapter 13

Is Your Hospital Breastfeeding Friendly?

It is critical that you assess the degree of breastfeeding support available at your birthing facility. It has been shown that nursing early and often is crucial to ultimate breastfeeding success. Since the majority of American mothers give birth in hospitals, that will the main focus of this chapter. Some outdated routines such as mother-infant separation, scheduled or timed feeds, and routine supplemental bottles (which have all been proven to decrease breastfeeding success) persist to varying degrees in most U.S. hospitals.

Your best bet is a hospital which has applied for a Certificate of Intent from the U.S. Committee for UNICEF for the Baby-Friendly Hospital Initiative (BFHI). BFHI is a research-based world standard with guidelines for maternity facilities to provide optimal breast-feeding support. Their *Ten Steps to Successful Breastfeeding* are as follows [comments on the rationale for some of these guidelines are in square brackets]:

1. Have a written breastfeeding policy which is regularly communicated to all health care staff.

2. Train all health care staff in the skills necessary to implement this policy. [Health care staff who have been trained in lactation

Excerpted from "If Breastfeeding Is So Wonderful, Why Aren't More Women Doing It?" by Alicia Dermer, M.D., I.B.C.L.C. ©1998–2000 by Joel R. Cooper, http://medicalreporter.health.org; reprinted with permission. Table excerpted from U.S. Department of Health and Human Services 2000 "Blueprint for Action on Breastfeeding," available at www.4woman.gov.

Table 13.1. Hospital Practices Which Influence Breastfeeding Initiation

Strongly Encouraging	Encouraging	Discouraging	Strongly Discouraging
Physical Cues			
baby put to breast immediately in delivery room	staff sensitivity to cultural norms and expectations of women	scheduled feedings regardless of mother's breastfeeding wishes	mother-infant separation at birth
baby not taken from mother after delivery			mother and infant housed on separate floors in postpartum period
women helped by staff to nurse baby in recovery room			mother separated from baby due to bilirubin problem
rooming-in; staff help with baby care in room, not only in nursery			no rooming-in policy
Verbal Communication			
staff initiates discussion re: woman's intention to breastfeed pre- and intrapartum	appropriate language skills of staff, teaching how to handle breast engorgement and nipple problems	staff instructs woman get good night's rest and miss a feeding	woman told to "take it easy," "get some rest," giving the impression that breastfeeding is effortful/ tiring
staff encourages and reinforces breast feeding immediately on labor and delivery	staff's own skills and comfort with the art of breastfeeding, time to teach woman on one-to-one basis	strict times allotted for breastfeeding regardless of mother/ baby's feeding cycle	woman told she doesn't "do it right;" staff interrupts her efforts, corrects her positions, etc.
staff discusses use of breast pump and realities of separation from baby			

Nonverbal Communication

pictures of woman breastfeeding	literature on breastfeeding in understandable terms	woman given infant formula kit and infant food literature
staff (doctors as well as nurses) give reinforcement for breastfeeding (respect, smiles, affirmation)	closed circuit TV show in hospital on breastfeeding	
nurse (or any attendant) making mother comfortable and helping to arrange baby at breast for nursing	pictures of woman bottle feeding	woman sees official-looking nurses authoritatively caring for babies by bottle feeding (leads to woman's insecurities re: own capability of care)
woman sees others breast-feeding in hospital	staff interrupts her breast-feeding session for lab tests, etc.	
	woman doesn't see others breastfeeding	

Experiential

if breastfeeding not immediately successful, staff continues to be supportive		previous failure with breastfeeding experience in hospital
previous success with breast-feeding experience in hospital		

77

management demonstrate a significant improvement in their practice.]

3. Inform all pregnant women of the benefits and management of breastfeeding. [Women who have had prenatal breast-feeding instruction have better breastfeeding outcomes.]

4. Help mothers to initiate breastfeeding within a half hour after birth. [In the U.S. BFHI, this reads "within an hour after birth." However, breastfeeding during the early alert period immediately after birth allows the baby to "imprint" on mother's nipple, and has been shown to increase breastfeeding success.]

5. Show mothers how to breastfeed, and how to maintain lactation if separated from their infants. [If the baby is not able to remove milk from the mother's breast, she needs to express the milk in order to keep up her milk supply.]

6. Give newborns no food or drink other than breastmilk unless medically necessary. [Formula is poorly digested and sits in baby's stomach much longer than mother's milk; a baby who is full of formula does not nurse often enough, and mother's milk supply drops. Also, even a single bottle of formula can predispose an allergy-prone baby to asthma, eczema, and allergies.]

7. Practice rooming-in to allow mothers and babies to remain together twenty-four hours a day. [Rooming-in mothers and babies get in tune with each other and have more chances to practice breastfeeding. This increased breastfeeding frequency ensures success.]

8. Encourage breastfeeding on demand. [When babies can regulate the timing and frequency of their feedings, rather than being scheduled or having the time on each breast limited, the mother's milk supply comes in much quicker.]

9. Give breastfeeding infants no artificial teats or pacifiers. [Artificial nipples promote a different sucking action from that required for breastfeeding. Some babies who have had bottles have difficulty learning to breastfeed. Pacifiers satisfy sucking needs, keeping some babies from going to the breast unless they are very hungry. This decreases mother's milk supply.]

10. Establish breastfeeding support groups and refer mothers to them after discharge.

Currently, over 300 hospitals in the U.S. have applied for a certificate of intent and are in the process of implementing the above guidelines. Fifteen hospitals and birthing facilities have now been certified "Baby Friendly". If you are lucky enough to deliver at one of these centers, you have a good chance of avoiding some of the early hospital practices which can interfere with your breastfeeding success.

If your hospital neither has a certificate of intent nor is certified, it may help you to take a few steps. First of all, discuss your concerns with your obstetrical care provider and your baby's doctor, and request that he/she be your advocate by writing explicit orders in line with the *Ten Steps*. Then, let hospital administration know of your wishes. Make up a written birth plan and make sure that it is known by the staff. Most importantly, enlist your own support people (e.g. baby's father, grandparents, designated labor coach) to advocate for you if you should be unable to insist on having your wishes followed. You may be too weak, drugged, or otherwise unable to insist that your baby be brought back to you from the nursery, but the father may well be able to do this. Even if you've had a Cesarean birth, as long as you and the baby are medically stable you should be able to nurse early and often. This would be another situation where your support people can intervene.

Of all the *Ten Steps*, the one which is most likely to help you and your baby get off to a good start is #7. If you room-in with your baby, you will get to know his/her early hunger cues such as rapid eye movements, sucking on hands, and rooting movements of the mouth, and then promptly put the baby to the breast. A mother whose baby is in the nursery must rely on the nurse to bring the baby, which usually occurs after the baby is long past these early hunger signs, when the baby has been screaming for several minutes, and is too upset from hunger and frustration to practice breastfeeding. Also, despite all well-meaning reassurances that the baby will be brought out in the middle of the night every time he/she is hungry, there are still nurses who give the baby bottles of formula either inadvertently or on purpose. Then the baby is brought to mom, stomach full of formula which sits there longer because it is so poorly digested, and is not interested in nursing. Mother's breasts are not being drained to signal more milk to be made, and mother feels rejected and loses self-confidence. Rooming in effectively prevents this. Don't be fooled into believing that leaving the baby in the nursery will ensure a good night's sleep. In one study, mothers whose babies were kept in the nursery were found not to sleep any better than those who roomed-in.

Another option available to some mothers is a free–standing midwife birthing center, which may be preferable if the pregnancy is not high risk and there is obstetrician back-up with a hospital nearby. These centers tend to provide natural birthing experiences and may be more conducive to breastfeeding success.

Chapter 14

How to Know a If Health Professional Is Not Supportive of Breastfeeding

Doctors agree that breastfeeding is best for newborns. But do doctors know enough about it to help new mothers get started? Researchers say many don't.

When physicians were surveyed about their knowledge of breastfeeding, they said that doctors-in-training aren't properly educated about the importance of breastfeeding. Many of them felt their training on breastfeeding was inadequate. For example, only about half of the doctors recalled a demonstration of breastfeeding during their medical training.

The researchers worry that if the young physicians don't understand breastfeeding they won't encourage their patients to try it and won't be able to help their patients if they have trouble breast feeding. Several of the surveyed physicians did not know how to recognize a woman who is physically unable to produce enough milk to breast feed. Fewer than five percent of women fall into that category.

Major pediatric and family medicine societies agree on the importance of breastfeeding. Other research has shown that breastfed babies tend to have fewer ear infections, respiratory tract infections, and bouts of diarrhea than bottle-fed babies.

From "Docs and Breastfeeding" © University of Texas Southwestern Medical Center at Dallas, updated 1998, used with permission. And excerpts from Handout #5 "How to Know a Health Professional Is Not Supportive of Breastfeeding," Jack Newman, M.D., F.R.C.P.C. Revised January 1998, reprinted with permission.

All health professionals say they are supportive of breastfeeding. But many are supportive only when breastfeeding is going well. As soon as breastfeeding, or anything in the life of the new mother is not perfect, too many advise weaning or supplementation. The following is a list of clues which help you judge whether or not a health professional is supportive of breastfeeding.

Warning Signs that Your Health Professional Is Not Supportive of Breastfeeding

She gives you formula samples or formula company literature when you are pregnant or after you have had the baby.

These samples and literature are inducements to use the product, and their distribution is called marketing. There is no evidence that any particular formula is better or worse than any other for the normal baby. The literature or videos accompanying samples are a means of subtly and not so subtly undermining breastfeeding and glorifying formula. Shouldn't you wonder why the health professional is not marketing breastfeeding?

She tells you that breastfeeding and bottle feeding are essentially the same.

Most bottle-fed babies grow up healthy and secure and not all breastfed babies grow up healthy and secure. However, this does not mean that breastfeeding and bottle feeding are essentially the same. Infant formula is a rough approximation of what we knew several years ago about breastmilk, which is in itself a rough approximation of something we are only beginning to get an inkling of and are constantly being surprised by. The differences have important health consequences. Certain elements in breastmilk are not in formula, even though we have known of their importance to the baby for several years. Breastfeeding is not the same as bottle feeding, it is a whole different relationship. A baby does not have to be breastfed to grow up happy, healthy, and secure, but it is an advantage.

She tells you that it is not necessary to feed the baby immediately after the birth since you will be tired and the baby is often not interested anyhow.

It isn't necessary, but it is very helpful. Babies can nurse while the mother is lying down or sleeping, though most mothers do not want to sleep at a moment such as this. Babies do not always show an interest in feeding immediately, but this is not a reason to prevent them from having the opportunity. Many babies latch on in the hour or two after delivery, and this is the time which is most conducive to getting started well, but they can't do it if they are separated from their mothers.

She tells you that there is no such thing as nipple confusion and you should start giving bottles early to your baby to make sure that the baby accepts a bottle nipple.

Why do you have to start giving bottles early if there is no such thing as nipple confusion? The artificial nipple has not been proved harmless to breastfeeding. It is often a combination of factors, including using an artificial nipple, which cause difficulties in the breastfeeding relationship.

She tells you that you must stop breastfeeding because you are sick, your baby is sick, you will be taking medicine, or you will have a medical test done.

There are occasional rare situations when breastfeeding cannot continue, but often when health professionals assume that the mother cannot continue they are wrong. The health professional who is supportive of breastfeeding will make efforts to find out how to avoid interruption of breastfeeding.

She is surprised to learn that your six-month-old baby is still breastfeeding.

In most of the world, breastfeeding to two or three years of age is common and normal.

She tells you that there is no value in breastmilk after the baby is six months or older.

Breastmilk is still milk with fat, protein, calories, and vitamins; and the antibodies and other elements which protect the baby against infections are still there, some in greater quantities than when the baby was younger. There is also still value in breastfeeding—it is a unique interaction between two people in love even without the milk.

She tells you that you must never allow your baby to fall asleep at the breast.

It is fine if a baby can also fall asleep without nursing, but one of the advantages of breastfeeding is that you have a handy way of putting your tired baby to sleep. Mothers around the world since the beginning of time have done just that. One of the great pleasures of parenthood is having a child fall asleep in your arms and feeling the warmth he gives off as sleep overcomes him. It is one of the pleasures of breastfeeding, both for the mother and probably also for the baby, when the baby falls asleep at the breast.

She tells you that you should not stay in the hospital to nurse your sick child because it is important you rest at home.

It is important that you rest, and the hospital which is supportive of breastfeeding will arrange it so that you can rest while you stay in the hospital to nurse your baby. Sick babies do not need breastfeeding less than a healthy baby, they need it more.

Part Three

The Early Weeks

Chapter 15

Beginning Breastfeeding in the Hospital

You have been given many helpful hints in the past months about how to take care of yourself and your new baby. This chapter helps you to focus on the important things about helping your baby learn to breastfeed. Keep the baby with you in your room so you will learn to tell when she is hungry. You will have many chances to practice breastfeeding.

Put baby to breast eight to twelve times every twenty-four hours that you are in the hospital. Nursing soon and often will help your milk come in faster. Hold your baby in a cradle position. The baby's neck is resting in the bend of your elbow. Turn your baby so you are tummy to tummy. Your baby's mouth should be at your breast.

Next, use your other arm to help your baby put his mouth over your nipple and areola. With your palm toward your chest, put your fingers below your breast and put your thumb on top. Gently squeeze a few drops of milk flow over your nipple and touch his lower lip. When he opens his mouth wide, put your breast into his mouth above his tongue. Then quickly pull him close so his mouth closes on the nipple and areola.

Keep the baby on the breast until he is done. He will either come off by himself or will move into a gentle, sleepy, "hanging out" type of suck. There is no magic number of minutes a baby should be at the breast. A sleepy baby is not necessarily a well-fed baby. Use these five

---

From the University of Iowa Healthbook (Virtual Hospital), www.vh.org. ©1992–1999, reprinted with permission of the University of Iowa.

behavioral cues to know when to awaken your baby more fully and begin breastfeeding:

1. Rapid eye movements under the eyelids

2. Sucking movements of the mouth and tongue

3. Hand to mouth movements

4. Body movements

5. Small sounds

This works better than waiting a set number of hours before attempting each feeding. Also, trying to wake a baby from a deep sleep will prove frustrating for both of you. Avoid covering the baby's hands with his undershirt cuffs or wrapping him in such away that his arms are pinned to his sides. This prevents him from sucking on his fist, which is comforting and also serves as a feeding cue.

If the baby is poky at the breast or falls asleep after a few sucks, use a method called "alternate massage" to help the baby keep sucking and take in a good deal of colostrum. Each time the baby pauses between sucking bursts, massage and compress your breast to get her started again. When she will no longer suck and swallow on the first side when you compress the breast, sit her up, burp her, and put her on the other breast. If she will not take the second side, she will cycle into a lighter sleep state in about forty-five to sixty minutes and can be given the second breast then.

Learn to tell when your baby is swallowing milk. Just because his jaw is moving does not necessarily mean he is getting milk. You can tell a baby is swallowing by:

*   Listening for a swallow after every one to four sucks

*   Listening for a puff of air from her nose following the swallow

*   Seeing or feeling his throat move with the swallow

*   Seeing or feeling the areola drawn into the baby's mouth as her jaw drops down

*   Seeing the back of the baby's head vibrate with the swallow

What If?

*   What if your baby will not breastfeed?

*   What if you cannot latch the baby to breast by yourself?

- What if you are having trouble telling whether the baby is swallowing?

- What if the baby has not breastfed two times in a row?

This is good time to ask your doctor, midwife, or your nurse for additional help and suggestions. Also make sure you have someone available to you who knows how to help you once you return home. You can always call your hospital or clinic for answers to your questions and concerns.

How Do You Know That Your Baby Is Getting Enough Milk?

1. Does the baby nurse eight or more times in twenty-four hours?

2. Does the baby have six to eight good wet diapers and three or more dirty diapers every day?

3. Does your baby seem content for one to two hours between most feedings?

4. Is your baby gaining at least one pound every month?

If the answers are YES, your baby is getting enough milk. Relax and enjoy breastfeeding your baby.

Remember growth spurts occur around two weeks, six weeks, and three months of age. You will find that your baby wants to nurse more frequently. This is your baby's way of making more milk. Let your baby feed often and you will have more milk in a day or two.

Chapter 16

Your Newborn

Babies are born wanting to suck, but feeling hungry and learning to eat are new for them. Many babies breastfeed easily. Other babies need help to get started.

It is a good idea to get your baby started feeding in the first hour or two after birth. Your baby will be wide awake right after birth. This is a good time to hold your baby close. It is also easier for the baby to learn how to breastfeed when she is alert. Tell your nurse that you want to breastfeed. Ask for help if you want it.

Feeding Your Baby

New babies need to eat often because they have small stomachs. Most babies nurse at least eight times every twenty-four hours for thirty to forty minutes each time. The first few days are a learning time for you and your baby.

Sleepy Baby

If your baby is sleepy, wake the baby every three hours during the day and once during the night. If you nurse at seven in the morning, nurse again by ten, even if you have to wake the baby. Wake your baby by talking close to the baby's face. Rub the baby's back, arms, legs,

An undated publication from North Carolina Department of Health and Human Services Nutri-NET Child Nutrition Information (http://wch.dhhs. state.nc.us). Reprinted with permission.

and tummy. Put a clean finger in the baby's mouth to get the baby sucking. Change the diaper. It may take about five minutes to wake your baby. You may need to do this before every feeding for a few days.

Once your baby starts gaining weight and wakes up regularly during the day for feedings, you can go to feeding on demand. That means the baby will let you know when it is time for a feeding. It is still okay to wake your baby if your breasts are feeling very full, or if you want to get the baby fed before doing something else.

One Breast or Both

Babies usually nurse from each breast at each feeding. Most babies need to burp when switched from one breast to the other. Sometimes, your baby may be too full to nurse from both breasts. If your baby nursed well and is acting full after one breast, that is okay. Just start the next feeding with the other breast.

If your baby falls asleep before finishing the first breast, wake the baby. Babies need to learn to nurse long enough to get full at each feeding.

If your baby stops sucking and swallowing after about fifteen minutes, but still wants to nurse, you will know the first breast is finished. You may also notice your breast soften during the feeding. Always be sure the baby finishes nursing the first breast before switching the baby to the other side. This way your baby will get the creamy part of the milk that comes at the end of the feeding. Cream has more calories which your baby needs to grow and feel full longer.

Growth Spurts

When your baby is seven to ten days old she will probably have a growth spurt. This may happen again at about three weeks. Your baby will want to nurse more often than usual. Even though your breasts may not feel full, let the baby nurse. In a few days you will be making more milk and the baby will nurse less often.

Bowel Movements

Your baby's bowel movements will change in the first few days. They will change from brown and sticky to watery and yellow. This tells you the baby is digesting breast milk. By the time the baby is four days old, you should see two to five yellow bowel movements a day. Some babies have a small stool with every feeding. As your baby gets older the number of bowel movements may decrease.

Crying or Fussy Baby

Crying is the only way your baby can call for help. If you just finished nursing, try other ways of comforting. The baby may need to burp, have a diaper change, or just need to be held. If you can not calm the baby, nurse again.

Sometimes it is hard to figure out why a baby is fussy. If your baby is crying a lot and wants to nurse more often than every two hours, the baby may be going through a growth spurt or may not be getting full at each feeding. Try holding your breast the whole time the baby nurses. This keeps the nipple far back in the baby's mouth so the milk can flow easily. Rub the baby's back and chest when the baby stops sucking. Keep doing this so the baby will nurse long enough to get full. Then the baby may be more content.

If your baby becomes very fussy and does not nurse well for two feedings, this may be a sign that the baby is sick. Call the baby's doctor or clinic. When a baby has an ear infection, thrush, or an upset stomach, sucking and swallowing may be painful.

Chapter 17

Taking Care of Yourself

Breast Care

Bras

If you wear a bra, dry your nipples before closing the flaps after feedings. Most women wear the same size bra at the end of pregnancy as they need while they are breastfeeding. If you want to buy new bras, wait until your baby is at least two weeks old and the early swelling is gone.

Washing

Wash your breasts with clear water once a day when you bathe. The small bumps on the areola make an oil that keeps the nipples clean and soft. Soap will wash away that oil.

Creams

Creams can block the natural oil your body makes. You do not need any cream around the nipples. If your nipples feel dry or if your nipples crack, rub breast milk on them to help them heal.

An undated publication from North Carolina Department of Health and Human Services Nutri-NET Child Nutrition Information (http://wch.dhhs. state.nc.us). Reprinted with permission.

Leaking Milk

During a feeding, the breast the baby is not nursing may start to leak. Press straight in on the nipple for several seconds to stop the leaking, or use a cup to collect milk for storing.

If you start to leak when you are not nursing, fold your arms across your chest and push in on your nipples for a few seconds. This will stop the milk flow.

You can wear breast pads in your bra if you need them. Change them whenever they are wet. Do not use pads with plastic liners. They may keep your nipples wet and that can make you sore. Many mothers never leak and do not need breast pads.

Some mothers find their breasts leak milk when they have sex. If this is a problem, try nursing right before, so your breasts are fairly empty.

Some mothers never leak milk. Most mothers leak less after the first few weeks of breastfeeding.

Nutrition, Exercise, and Rest

Nutrition

As a breastfeeding mother you do not need to watch what you eat and drink the way you may have when you were pregnant. Your body will change naturally to make you hungrier and thirstier. If you eat enough to feel full and drink enough so you are not thirsty, your milk will have everything your baby needs to grow and be healthy.

You will feel your best if you eat a balanced diet whether you are breastfeeding or not. Fruits and vegetables; cereals and grains; dairy products; and protein foods like dried beans, peanut butter, and meats are needed for good health. If there are days when you do not eat right, you will still make healthy milk.

You do not need to drink a special amount because you are breastfeeding. If your urine is dark and smells strong, or if you are constipated, drink more liquid. Eating soups will also add liquid to your diet.

Caffeine will be in your breast milk if you drink a lot of fluids with caffeine, like coffee, tea, or soft drinks. Caffeine causes some babies to be very active and have trouble sleeping. If your baby is fussy, cut back on drinks with caffeine in them.

Weight Loss

Many breastfeeding mothers can lose weight easily. Making breast milk uses calories. If you want to lose weight:

- Drink skim or low-fat milk instead of whole milk.

- Cut down on sweets like cake, cookies, and candy.

- Drink fruit juice, water, or club soda instead of sweet tea and soda.

- Choose baked or broiled foods instead of fried foods.

- Snack on fresh fruit, raw vegetables, or plain popcorn.

- Limit greasy foods like bacon, sausage, fatback, gravy, donuts, and chips.

- Take a walk with your baby every day.

- Talk with the nutritionist or your doctor if you have questions about losing weight while you are breastfeeding.

Exercise

You can run, do aerobics, or play sports while you are breastfeeding. If you nurse just before exercising, your breasts will not be as full and you will be more comfortable. You may find that you feel better if you are wearing a bra with good support.

Rest

Many mothers get tired taking care of a new baby. Lying down to nurse is one way to rest. Try not to do everything at first. Having visitors and cleaning can wait. When people want to help, let them cook, get groceries, do laundry or play with your other children while you and your baby rest together.

It is not a good idea for the baby to have a bottle while you sleep. Your full breasts will hurt and wake you up. Your breasts may get too hard for the baby to nurse easily.

If someone wants to help with the baby, they can give the baby a bath, change the diapers, or take the baby for a walk.

Smoking, Alcohol, and Drugs

Smoking

If you smoke, the health of you and your baby is at risk. Babies and young children raised in homes with cigarette smoke get ear infections and colds more often. Now may be a good time to think about quitting. If you cannot quit smoking, you can still breastfeed.

Nicotine can slow your milk let-down and production. Quit smoking or smoke after a feeding instead of before or during a feeding.

Nicotine in breastmilk may cause some babies to have gas and be fussy. Quit smoking or cut back on the number of cigarettes you smoke each day.

Never smoke in the same room as a baby. Smoke is bad for all babies' lungs.

Alcohol

The alcohol in beer, wine, and liquor goes into your milk and to your baby. Breastfeeding mothers should have no more than one beer, one glass of wine, or one mixed drink in a day. If you want a drink, time it so you are drinking just after a breastfeeding.

Medicines

Medicines can go through your milk to the baby. Check with the baby's doctor before taking any, even over-the-counter medicines. Tell the doctor you are breastfeeding. If you are sick and need medicine, the doctor can usually find a safe one for you to take and continue breastfeeding.

Street Drugs

Street drugs go through your milk to your baby. They are dangerous for both you and your baby. If you are using drugs, get help to stop. If you are going to use street drugs, DO NOT BREASTFEED.

Sex and Birth Control

Having a baby may make you feel differently about sex. Some women feel sexier, but some women are not interested in sex at all for awhile. It is normal to have changing feelings. When you are ready for sex again, there are some things you will want to know:

- Some women leak milk when they have sex. If you nurse the baby first, your breasts will not be as full, and this may not happen as much. It is okay for your partner to play with your breasts. You will still have milk for the next feeding.

- Your vagina (birth canal) may be dry after your baby is born. Using extra contraceptive foam or a special lubricant like K-Y

Jelly or Lubrifax may help. If using condoms, do not use a petroleum-based lubricant like Vaseline.

• Many women with new babies do not feel ready for another pregnancy. Waiting at least a year before you become pregnant again may be better for your health. Waiting may also improve your chance of having a healthy baby.

• You can get pregnant while breastfeeding. It is important to use a birth control method if you do not want to get pregnant.

Chapter 18

Postpartum Depression

Are Changes in Mood Common after Childbirth?

After having a baby, many women have mood swings. One minute they feel happy, the next minute they start to cry. They may feel a little depressed, have a hard time concentrating, lose their appetite, or find that they can't sleep well even when the baby is asleep. These symptoms usually start about three to four days after delivery and may last several days.

If you're a new mother and have any of these symptoms, you have what is called the baby blues. The blues are considered a normal part of early motherhood and usually go away within 10 days after delivery. However, some women have worse symptoms or symptoms that last longer. This is called postpartum depression.

What Is Postpartum Depression?

Postpartum depression is an illness, like diabetes or heart disease. It can be treated with therapy, support networks, and medicines such as antidepressants. Here are some symptoms of postpartum depression:

- Loss of interest or pleasure in life.

- Loss of appetite.
- Less energy and motivation to do things.
- A hard time falling asleep or staying asleep.
- Sleeping more than usual.
- Increased crying or tearfulness.
- Feeling worthless, hopeless, or overly guilty.
- Feeling restless, irritable, or anxious.
- Unexplained weight loss or gain.
- Feeling like life isn't worth living.
- Having thoughts about hurting yourself.
- Worrying about hurting your baby.

Although many women get depressed right after childbirth, some women don't feel down until several weeks or months later. Depression that occurs within six months of childbirth may be postpartum depression.

Who Gets Postpartum Depression?

Postpartum depression is more likely if you had any of the following:

- Previous postpartum depression.
- Depression not related to pregnancy.
- Severe premenstrual syndrome (PMS).
- A difficult marriage.
- Few family members or friends to talk to or depend on.
- Stressful life events during the pregnancy or after the childbirth.

Why Do Women Get Postpartum Depression?

The exact cause isn't known. Hormone levels change during pregnancy and right after childbirth. Those hormone changes may produce chemical changes in the brain that play a part in causing depression.

Feeling depressed doesn't mean that you're a bad person, or that you did something wrong, or that you brought this on yourself.

How Long Does Postpartum Depression Last?

It's hard to say. Some women feel better within a few weeks, but others feel depressed or "not themselves" for many months. Women who have more severe symptoms of depression or who have had depression in the past may take longer to get well. Just remember that help is available and that you can get better.

What Kinds of Treatments Help with Postpartum Depression?

Postpartum depression is treated much like any other depression. Support, counseling ("talk therapy"), and medicines can help.

If I'm Breastfeeding, Can I Take an Antidepressant?

If you take an antidepressant medicine, it will go into your breastmilk. Talk to your doctor about the risks of taking an antidepressant while breastfeeding. Your doctor can decide which medicine may be best for you to use while nursing your baby.

What Can I Do to Help Myself?

If you have given birth recently and are feeling sad, blue, anxious, irritable, tired, or have any of the other symptoms mentioned here, remember that many other women have had the same experience. You're not "losing your mind" or "going crazy" and you shouldn't feel that you just have to suffer. Here are some things you can do that other mothers with postpartum depression have found helpful:

- Find someone to talk to, and tell that person about your feelings.

- Get in touch with people who can help you with child care, household chores, and errands. This social support network will help you find time for yourself so you can rest.

- Find time to do something for yourself, even if it's only fifteen minutes a day.

- Try reading, exercising (walking is good for you and easy to do), taking a bath, or meditating.

- Keep a diary. Every day, write down your emotions and feelings as a way of "letting it all out." Once you begin to feel better, you can go back and reread your diary—this will help you see how much better you are.

- Even if you can only get one thing done in any given day, this is a step in the right direction. There may be days when you can't get anything done. Try not to get angry with yourself when this happens.

- It's OK to feel overwhelmed. Childbirth brings many changes, and parenting is challenging. When you're not feeling like yourself, these changes can seem like too much to cope with.

- You're not expected to be a "supermom." Be honest about how much you can do, and ask other people to help you.

- Find a support group in your area or contact one of the organizations listed below. They can put you in touch with people near you who have experience with postpartum depression.

- Talk with your doctor about how you feel. He or she may offer counseling and/or medicines that can help.

Postpartum Depression Resources

The following organizations can help you find a support group:

Postpartum Support International
927 N. Kellogg
Santa Barbara, CA 93111
Phone: 805-967-7636
Fax: 805-967-0608
Website: www.chss.iup.edu/postpartum

Postpartum Education for Parents
P.O. Box 6154
Santa Barbara, CA 93160
Website: www.sbpep.org

Part Four

Breastfeeding as a Baby Grows

Chapter 19

Is My Baby Getting Enough Milk?

Breastfeeding mothers frequently ask how to know their babies are getting enough milk. The breast is not the bottle, and it is not possible to hold the breast up to the light to see how many ounces or milliliters of milk the baby drank. Our number-obsessed society makes it difficult for some mothers to accept not seeing exactly how much milk the baby receives. However, there are ways of knowing that the baby is getting enough. In the long run, weight gain is the best indication whether the baby is getting enough, but rules about weight gain appropriate for bottle-fed babies may not be appropriate for breastfed babies.

Ways of Knowing Your Baby Is Getting Enough Milk

Characteristic Sucking

A baby who is obtaining lots of milk at the breast sucks in a very characteristic way. The baby generally opens his mouth fairly wide as he sucks and the rhythm is slow and steady. His lips are turned out. At the maximum opening of his mouth, there is a perceptible pause which you can see if you watch his chin. Then, the baby closes his mouth again. This pause does not refer to the pause between suckles, but rather to the pause during one suckle as the baby opens his mouth to its maximum. Each one of these pauses corresponds to a mouthful

Handout 4, "Is My Baby Getting Enough?" by Jack Newman M.D., F.R.C.P.C., revised 1998. Reprinted with permission.

of milk and the longer the pause, the more milk the baby got. At times, the baby can even be heard to be swallowing, and this is perhaps reassuring, but the baby can be getting lots of milk without making noise. Usually, the baby's suckle will change during the feeding so that the above type of suck will alternate with sucks that could be described as "nibbling." This is normal. The baby who suckles as described above, with several minutes of pausing type sucks at each feeding, and then comes off the breast satisfied is getting enough. The baby who nibbles only, or has the drinking type of suckle for a short period of time only, is probably not. This is the best way of knowing the baby is getting enough. This type of suckling can be seen on the very first day of life, though it is not as obvious as later when the mother has lots more milk.

Bowel Movements

For the first few days after delivery, the baby passes meconium, a dark green, almost black, substance. Meconium accumulates in the baby's gut during pregnancy. Meconium is passed during the first few days, and by the third day, the bowel movements start becoming lighter as more breastmilk is taken. Usually by the fifth day, the bowel movements have taken on the appearance of the normal breastmilk stool. The normal breastmilk stool is pasty to watery, mustard colored, and usually has little odor. However, bowel movements may vary considerably from this description. They may be green or orange, may contain curds or mucus, or may resemble shaving lotion in consistency (from air bubbles). The variation in color does not mean something is wrong. A baby who is breastfeeding only, and is starting to have bowel movements which are becoming lighter by day three of life, is doing well.

Monitoring the frequency and quantity of bowel motions is one of the best ways of knowing if the baby is getting enough milk. After the first three to four days, the baby should have increasing bowel movements so that by the end of the first week he should be passing at least 2-3 substantial yellow stools each day. In addition, many infants have a stained diaper with almost each feeding. A baby who is still passing meconium on the fifth day should be seen at the clinic the same day. A baby who is passing only brown bowel movements is probably not getting enough, but this is not yet definite.

Any baby between five and twenty-one days of age who does not pass at least one substantial bowel movement within a 24 hour period should be seen at the breastfeeding clinic the same day. Generally, small infrequent bowel movements during this time period means insufficient intake. There are definite exceptions and everything may be fine, but it is better to check.

Some breastfed babies, after the first three to four weeks of life, may suddenly change their stool pattern from many each day to one every three days or even less. Some babies have gone as long as fifteen days or more without a bowel movement. As long as the baby is otherwise well, and the stool is the usual pasty or soft, yellow movement, this is not constipation and is of no concern.

Urination

With six soaking-wet (not just wet) diapers in a twenty-four hour period after about four to five days of life, you can be sure that the baby is getting a lot of milk. Unfortunately, the new super-dry disposable diapers often do indeed feel dry even when full of urine, but when soaked with urine they are heavy. It should be obvious that this indication of milk intake does not apply if you are giving the baby extra water (which is unnecessary for breastfed babies). The baby's urine should be clear as water after the first few days, though an occasional darker urine is not of concern.

The Following Are NOT Good Ways of Knowing Your Baby Is Getting Enough Milk

1. Your breasts do not feel full. After the first few days or weeks, it is usual for most mothers not to feel full. Your body adjusts to your baby's requirements. This change may occur quite suddenly. Some mothers breastfeeding perfectly well never feel engorged or full.

2. The baby sleeps through the night. Not necessarily. A baby who is sleeping through the night at ten days of age may, in fact, not be getting enough milk. A baby who is too sleepy and has to be awakened for feeds or who is "too good" may not be getting enough milk. There are many exceptions, but get help quickly.

3. The baby cries after feeding. Although the baby may cry after feeding because of hunger, there are also many other reasons for crying. Do not limit feeding times.

4. The baby feeds often and/or for a long time. For one mother every three hours or so feedings may be often; for another,

three hours or so may be a long period between feeds. For one a feeding that lasts for thirty minutes is a long feeding; for another it is a short one. There are no rules how often or for how long a baby should nurse. Remember, a baby may be on the breast for 2 hours, but if he is actually breastfeeding (open-pause-close type of sucking) for only 2 minutes, he will come off the breast hungry. If the baby falls asleep quickly at the breast, you can compress the breast to continue the flow of milk. Contact the breastfeeding clinic with any concerns, but wait to start supplementing.

5. You can only express a small amount of milk. This means nothing and should not influence you. Therefore, you should not pump your breasts "just to know." Most mothers have plenty of milk. The problem is usually that the baby is not getting the milk that is there because he is latched on poorly, or because his suckle is ineffective, or both. These problems can often be fixed easily.

6. The baby will take a bottle after feeding. This does not necessarily mean that the baby is still hungry. This is not a good test, as bottles may interfere with breastfeeding.

7. The five-week-old baby is suddenly pulling away from the breast but still seems hungry. This does not mean your milk has "dried up" or decreased. During the first few weeks of life, babies often fall asleep at the breast when the flow of milk slows down even if they have not had their fill. When they are older (four to six weeks of age), they are no longer content to fall asleep, but rather start to pull away or get upset. The milk supply has not changed; the baby has. Compress the breast to increase flow.

Chapter 20

Using Bottles

First of all, obtain reliable information. Avoid formula-sponsored materials, which may have some accurate information but may omit important information or imply that supplementation with formula or eventual weaning to formula are desirable or inevitable. For example, formula-sponsored breastfeeding pamphlets do not state unequivocally that the American Academy of Pediatrics recommends breastfeeding for the full first year of life, exclusively for the first 6 months. Instead, there are words such as "breastfeed for as long as possible..." More importantly, although cow's milk protein and soy protein are the two most common allergy-causing substances in babies, there is no mention of the importance to families with histories of asthma, eczema, or allergies to breastfeed exclusively to avoid formula supplements to prevent sensitization of the baby to these proteins.

Although some formula literature now recommends waiting to introduce a bottle until at least 3 to 4 weeks, the implication is that the bottle will inevitably be introduced. In fact, bottle feeding (even with mother's milk) is not always desirable or necessary. Mothers who breastfeed according to the AAP recommendations may never need to introduce a bottle at all, as they can start the baby on cup feeds at

This document includes text from: "Using Bottles," undated, North Carolina Department of Health and Human Services Nutri-NET Child Nutrition Information (http://wch.dhhs.state.nc.us); reprinted with permission. And excerpts from "If Breastfeeding Is So Wonderful, Why Aren't More Women Doing It?" by Alicia Dermer, M.D., I.B.C.L.C. ©1998–2000 by Joel R. Cooper, http://medicalreporter.health.org; reprinted with permission.

111

six months and continue nursing. Even before six months, if the baby needs to be fed while mom is away, there are alternative feeding methods (e.g. spoons, medicine cups, medicine droppers or syringes, supplemental feeding tube devices) that can be used instead of bottles. Nipple preference (also known as nipple confusion) is most likely to occur while a baby is first learning to nurse, but breast refusal can occur at any age in a child who has been getting a lot of bottles. A baby's refusal to take a bottle is a remediable problem, whereas a baby unable to breastfeed because bottles were introduced too early may spell the end of the breastfeeding relationship.

So should you never use a bottle? Well, never say never. There are certainly situations in which bottles are fine. Some mothers never use bottles, but if you want to use them, it is best to wait at least four weeks to give the baby time to learn how to breastfeed well and to give your breasts time to get used to making milk. Once your baby is used to nursing, you can give bottles for some feedings without confusing your baby.

Some babies need to try a couple of times before they learn to take a bottle. If you try a bottle when your baby is very hungry, the baby may be too upset to learn how to use it.

Most babies do well with a regular nipple. Using a short, flat-ended nipple teaches some babies to bite during feedings. Try one type of nipple several times before switching to another type.

Hand Expressing and Pumping

Learning to express or pump milk takes practice. Do not worry if you only get a little milk. Many mothers get less than an ounce each time. With practice, you will be able to express more. You can get milk to use in a bottle by hand expressing, using a hand pump, or using a small electric pump. Wash your hands first.

Hand Expressing

Start by gently rubbing your breasts in small circles (the size of quarters). Rub all around the breast, starting at your chest and working toward your nipple.

Hold your breast in your fingers with your thumb on top. Push straight back toward your chest. Gently bring your thumb and forefinger together. Do not pinch the nipple. It may take several minutes to get the milk to flow. Keep moving your hand around your breast until you have softened all parts.

Using a Breast Pump

Follow the directions for the breast pump you have. Just like the baby does a suck and then a swallow, the pump should do a pull and then a release.

Storing Your Milk

The first time you hand express or pump, put the milk in a clean glass or plastic bottle or disposable bottle liners. Keep adding to the bottle until you have the amount you need. If your baby weighs less than ten pounds, put 2–3 ounces in a bottle. Once your baby weighs more than 10 pounds, make each bottle 4–6 ounces.

Store milk you will use within 48 hours in the refrigerator. To keep it longer, put it in the freezer. Thaw frozen milk when you are ready to use it. Put the bottle of breastmilk in a bowl of warm water. It will warm quickly. DO NOT WARM MILK IN A MICROWAVE OVEN. The milk can get too hot and burn the baby's mouth.

Using Infant Formula

You can breastfeed at some feedings and give infant formula at other feedings. It is best to wait until your baby is four or more weeks old and your milk supply is established before giving formula. The more formula you use, the less breast milk you make.

Your baby will grow on any of the major brands of iron-fortified formula.

Infant formula comes in three forms:

- Concentrated formula must be mixed with water in batches.

- Powdered formula can be mixed with water one bottle at a time or in batches.

- Ready-to-use formula does not need water added.

- Powdered formula is the most convenient for breastfeeding mothers because one bottle can be mixed at a time.

Chapter 21

Adding Solids

The energy and nutrient needs of the newborn to six-month-old infant are well met by breastmilk or commercial infant formula plus a fluoride supplement. By age six months, the infant needs an additional source of carbohydrate and more of vitamins A and C than provided in a milk-based diet alone.

Developmentally, the six-month-old is ready to sit upright with support, observe a spoon with food coming towards his mouth, open his mouth when ready for the food, and move the food from the spoon to a swallow. The six-month-old is also able to communicate his rejection of the food. The digestive system is mature enough to handle new foods. The younger infant is not developmentally able to do these things and is therefore not ready to be fed solid foods.

The first solid food introduced is usually iron-fortified infant rice cereal mixed with breastmilk or formula. Very few people are allergic to rice and it is easily digested, so it makes an excellent choice for a first food. Barley cereal is also an appropriate early solid. Start with just a tablespoon or so of cereal and a few teaspoons of breastmilk or formula. This is a new experience and it may take a few feedings before baby is ready for a quantity of cereal.

Feed baby in an upright position. Use rolled up towels or receiving blankets in a high chair if the infant needs additional support, or have one adult hold the infant while another offers the food to baby.

"Adding Solid Foods," an undated publication of the University of Rhode Island Cooperative Extension Expanded Food and Nutrition Program (EFNEP), www.uri.edu. Reprinted with permission.

115

Do not try to feed the baby in a semi-reclined position such as an infant carrier or car seat. It is very difficult for her to swallow while reclining and difficult to see the spoon as it comes toward her mouth. It is important that the infant be able to see the spoon coming towards her mouth so that she can open her mouth in anticipation. Do not force the spoon between closed lips as this turns feeding into an unpleasant experience and can cause many feeding problems later on. Use an infant size spoon. Many babies prefer a plastic or rubber-coated spoon—cold metal can be an unpleasant experience.

The baby who is developmentally ready for solids will learn to eagerly anticipate the full spoon coming towards his mouth and will be open and ready by the time it gets there. A baby who is reluctant to open and fusses and complains when the parent tries feeding for the first time may not be ready—wait a few days and then offer the food again.

Do not put infant cereal or any other solid into a bottle or infant feeder. It will interfere with the child's natural ability to obtain the appropriate amount of energy from the milk feeds. It is simply force feeding and inappropriate.

Once the infant is developmentally ready for solids, the parents need to be ready to change quickly. Infants are capable of very fast and rapid transitions from one ability to the next during the next few months. Parents need to be ready for those changes. Allow the child to take the lead as this chewing and swallowing ability progress. Learn to understand the child's nonverbal communications and relax.

After the child has done well with infant cereal for several weeks, pureed or strained fruits or vegetables may be added to the diet. Experts do not agree on whether to add fruits first or vegetables first, and it probably does not matter. But babies do have an innate preference for a sweet taste, so start with sweeter vegetables such as squash and sweet potatoes. Purchased infant foods or those made at home may be used. Baby does not need added sugar or salt. If home prepared foods are used, careful sanitation practices should be observed. Wait three to five days between each new food offered to make sure that there is not problem with a food allergy.

Watch baby's jaw as he is offered foods. When an up and down munching motion begins to be apparent, pureed meats, beans, cooked egg yolk, tofu, cottage cheese, and plain yogurt may be added to the diet.

Chapter 22

Vitamin and Fluoride Supplements

According to La Leche League's *The Womanly Art of Breastfeeding*, if a breastfeeding mother is getting an adequate supply of vitamins in her diet, then her milk will contain adequate nutrients in the perfect balance for her baby. If your baby is healthy and doing well, there is no need for vitamins, iron, or other supplements in the early months. Furthermore, many mothers have found that vitamin or fluoride supplements can cause fussiness and/or colic in their infants.

What about Vitamin D?

This nutrient is only available in small quantities in human milk. However, if just a small patch of your baby's skin is exposed to sunlight for just a few minutes each day, this will provide plenty of Vitamin D for most babies. If you live in a severe climate and go without any exposure to sunlight for months, or if you wear clothing that protects the skin from all sunlight, your baby may need a vitamin D supplement. La Leche League International (LLLI)'s *The Breastfeeding Answer Book* also notes that dark-skinned mothers and babies may need additional vitamin D.

What about Iron?

Human milk contains less iron than cow's milk. However, according to *The Breastfeeding Answer Book*, the iron in human milk is better absorbed by the human baby than is the iron in cow's milk or iron-fortified formula. The full-term, healthy baby usually has no need of additional iron until about the middle of his first year, around the time he starts taking solids. Then, it is easy to offer the baby foods which are naturally rich in iron.

What about Fluoride?

The American Academy of Pediatrics recommended in its 1995 policy statement that babies younger than six months should NOT receive fluoride supplements, and that babies older than six months receive supplements only if they live in an area where the drinking water contains less than 0.3 ppm of fluoride.

What about Vitamin B12?

Mothers on strict vegetarian diets excluding meat, fish, and dairy products may be deficient in this nutrient, although this is not common in North America. If a mother is deficient in this or another nutrient, she may find that improving her diet or taking supplements herself is as effective or more effective than giving them directly to the baby.

Chapter 23

Your One- to Six-Month-Old Baby

Some babies become very interested in what is happening around them at 2–3 months. They will stop nursing to look and then want to nurse again very soon. Feed the baby in a quiet room for a few days or use a teddy bear, doll, or blanket to block the baby's view. Then your baby will get used to nursing long enough to get full.

Feeding Your Baby

Most young babies need to eat about every three hours during the day and about every four hours at night. Babies also begin to nurse faster, so feedings may not take as long. As your baby grows, the time between feedings gets longer. The baby is usually able to sleep a little longer at night.

Babies need to suck. A baby who sucks on a thumb or pacifier between feedings and is having six wet diapers and regular bowel movements is probably not hungry. Many babies just like to suck. Do not worry if your baby seems to want to suck between feedings.

Night Feedings

During the night, most babies wake up less often than they do during the day. When your baby stirs and makes sounds, it might be

An undated publication from North Carolina Department of Health and Human Services Nutri-NET Child Nutrition Information (http://wch.dhhs.state.nc.us). Reprinted with permission.

119

time for a feeding. You can wait a few minutes to see if the baby goes back to sleep. If the baby stirs a lot or your breasts feel full and heavy, then it probably is time to feed.

As babies get older, they usually will go for longer times between feedings. Your body gets used to the longer times between feedings.

Starting Solid Foods

Between 4 and 6 months, your baby will show signs that he is ready for cereal. One sign is that your baby will be able to hold his head steady and sit with support. Another sign is up and down tongue movements which allow the baby to take cereal from a spoon and swallow easily. A baby who "spits" the cereal out when spoon fed may not be ready for solid foods. Breastfeed your baby before offering solid food. Your milk should still be your baby's main food.

Growth

Weight Gain

Your baby is probably getting enough if he is nursing well, is content after feeding, and is gaining weight. Most babies gain seven ounces every week until they double their birth weight. If your baby gains faster that is okay.

Growth Spurts

Babies need more milk as they grow. Your baby will want to nurse about twice as often as usual during a growth spurt. Growth spurts usually come when the baby is about seven to ten days, three weeks, six weeks, three months, and six months (or a little earlier). A baby who has been feeding about every three hours will want to eat every hour and a half. Even though your breasts do not feel full, let the baby nurse. You will know milk is there when you hear the baby swallow. After a day or two of feeding your baby very often, you will be making more milk at each feeding. Your baby will then go back to nursing less often.

Special Tips

- Few babies get hungry by the clock. Sometimes, your baby may be hungry soon after a feeding. When nothing else comforts the baby, nurse again.

- Babies like to be held and to be with people even when they are not eating. They like to see, hear, and learn from the world around them. Some mothers like to use front packs or baby slings to carry their babies close and still have a free hand. Your baby may also enjoy being in a swing sometimes.

- Your baby needs breast milk to grow well. Babies who drink water and eat other things when they are small may get too full and not want as much milk.

- Babies do not need anything but breastmilk for the first four to six months of life. Babies do not sleep better or grow faster if they have cereal or juice when they are small.

Chapter 24

Your Six- to Twelve-Month-Old Baby

Your baby will probably have doubled her birth weight by now. Your milk should still be your baby's main food, but she will start to eat more solid foods as she gets older. Your baby is ready to start drinking from a cup. Some of the liquid may dribble from the sides of the baby's mouth. Be ready; put a bib or cloth over the baby's clothes.

Feeding Your Baby

As your baby gets older, the time between breastfeedings will get longer. Your baby may not want to nurse at mealtimes. She will slowly start to eat more solid foods and nurse less often. Some babies continue to nurse about thirty minutes at each feeding and others nurse more quickly.

Sometimes your baby will want to eat a lot of solid foods. This is probably a growth spurt. Instead of nursing more, the baby is eating solid foods to meet her needs.

Sometimes your baby will want to nurse a lot and not want solid foods. These times may be when your baby is teething, not feeling well, or has just been given a shot. Offer the baby meals as usual, but then nurse if that is all the baby wants for a day or two.

An undated publication from North Carolina Department of Health and Human Services Nutri-NET Child Nutrition Information (http://wch.dhhs.state.nc.us). Reprinted with permission.

Using a Cup

Learning to drink from a cup is a new skill. Start with just a little in the cup at first. Offer sips of water, juice, or breastmilk from the cup. While a cup with a spout may help avoid spills, it does not help the baby to learn about drinking from a cup or glass.

Introducing New Foods

Once your baby is eating cereal from a spoon and swallowing easily, you may begin to add other foods to the baby's diet. Try only one new food at a time. Always wait three days before adding another food. This way, if your baby gets diarrhea, a rash, or other problem, you will know what food to stop.

Teething

Teething has probably started. Some babies do not want to nurse very much when they are cutting teeth because their gums hurt. Other babies want to nurse a lot because they do not feel good. Each baby is different. If your baby's gums seem to hurt, you can crush an ice cube in a clean washcloth and hold it while the baby chews or use a cold soft teething ring. The cold may help the gums feel better so your baby can nurse.

Nursing babies cannot get milk if they bite. Biting will pinch the nipple shut. When the baby is nursing, the tongue covers the lower gum. If your baby's tongue slips back and the baby starts to bite, you can stop the feeding. Your baby will quickly learn not to bite.

Special Tips

- Begin teaching your baby how to drink from a cup. Be prepared for spills.

- If your baby has trouble nursing because she is cutting teeth, you can crush an ice cube in a clean washcloth and hold it while the baby chews. The cold may make the gums feel better so your baby can nurse.

- As your baby begins eating more solid foods, the time between breastfeedings will get longer.

Chapter 25

Breastfeeding in Public

There's no need to stay at home just because you're breastfeeding. Mothers nurse their babies anywhere and everywhere, and you can learn to do this, too.

Discreet Breastfeeding

Breastfeeding at home in the first weeks postpartum includes lots of skin-to-skin contact with baby and lots of "letting it all hang out." Nursing at the mall, the museum, or your mother-in-law's house is going to require a different approach. There's really nothing wrong with exposing a breast so that a baby can nurse, but in most social situations most people are more comfortable when mothers nurse discreetly. Good manners suggest that you should take the feelings of others into account, but of course, your first consideration will be your baby. When he's hungry or in need of comfort, he wants the breast!

Tips for Breastfeeding Anytime, Anywhere

Some careful strategizing can make breastfeeding away from home seem like a simple and natural thing to do. Here are some tips on what to wear, how to get baby started, how to teach baby good nursing manners, where to nurse, what to do if someone hassles you, and how to help yourself and others feel more comfortable. Don't forget to practice discreet nursing at home first!

What to Wear

Simple, accessible clothing is the key to nursing in public. Wear clothes that make it easier to nurse discreetly.

- Two-piece outfits with loose tops are the best. You can lift the shirt from the bottom so the baby can get at the breast. The rest of the fabric will drape around the baby's head to cover any exposed skin.

- If you're wearing a shirt or blouse that buttons, unbutton it from the bottom up, rather than from the top down.

- Think of nursing in terms of snuggling your baby under your clothes rather than getting your breast out.

- A loose jacket or cardigan sweater can provide extra coverage for your middle.

- Drape a lightweight blanket or shawl over your shoulder and over baby as you nurse.

- An old T-shirt worn under a sweater or another shirt can provide extra coverage and protect your middle from icy drafts. Cut slits in the T-shirt at breast level. When you lift the outer shirt, the T-shirt stays in place.

- A baby sling is a real boon to discreet nursing. You can stroll through department stores or play with a toddler in the park while keeping baby latched on behind the fabric of the sling.

- Wear a large T-shirt over your swimsuit for discreet nursing at the beach. Or look for swimsuits made especially for breastfeeding women.

- If you yearn to wear dresses, look for special styles for nursing mothers with hidden openings at the breast. These are available from catalogs and can sometimes be found in maternity shops or online.

- Nursing bras with cups that are easy to unfasten with one hand can make it easy to get your baby started at the breast, but refastening bra cups often requires two hands. You might have to wait to do this until you have a private moment, a reason to avoid clingy or sheer tops when you're out with baby.

- Prints and loose styles camouflage leaking and spit-up stains.

How to Get Started

- One of the best ways to avoid drawing a lot of attention to yourself and your nursing baby is to be alert to your baby's hunger cues and feed him before he is howling. He'll latch on more easily, and you won't have lots of people scowling at you while you try to stop the noise.

- Expect that you will feed your baby while you're out at the mall or visiting friends. Don't nurse as a last resort, when all your attempts to distract your baby have failed.

- The breast may be exposed during the brief moment it takes for your little one to latch on. This is more of a problem with young babies than for experienced nursers. You can turn your back to the rest of the room while you get him started, or briefly go into another room and return once baby is latched on and blankets and clothing are discreetly arranged. Or, drape a blanket over your breast, arm, and baby during latch-on.

- Probably the easiest solution to this problem is to use a baby sling to carry your baby when you are out in public. When baby wants to nurse, pull up the fabric to cover your breast while baby is getting started.

- If you're sitting on a bench or a chair without arms, use your diaper bag, a folded sweater or coat, or something else in your lap to bring the baby up to breast level while you nurse. You'll enjoy your outing more if you don't go home with sore nipples or a cramp in your arm or back caused by poor positioning at the breast.

Teaching Your Baby Good Manners

- Remember, baby's head provides the crucial cover-up while she's at the breast. Keep an eye on your baby while she's nursing if she's the kind who likes to pop off and smile up at you from time to time. Be prepared to flip your shirt down during these tender moments.

- If you have a baby who loves to push your sweater up to your collarbone, try holding that free baby hand in yours while nursing in public places.

- As your baby gets older, teach her good nursing manners when you're nursing at home. Climbing around on your lap while nursing may seem okay on your living room sofa, but you probably won't appreciate this behavior at the family reunion.

Where to Nurse in Public

Here are some strategies for different locations:

- Choose an out-of-the-way place to nurse your baby, if possible, and if this really matters to you.

- In a restaurant, ask to be seated in a booth at the side of the room, rather than in the middle of everything. Sitting with your back to the room gives you more privacy.

- At the mall, look for a seating area with nooks and crannies or plants if you don't want to nurse in front of everyone who may be passing by. Or choose a comfortable place to sit down where you can people-watch while you nurse.

- Stop for a snack and nurse in a corner of the restaurant.

- If a store is not too busy, go ahead and use a fitting room.

- Nursing in church is a real hurdle for some women. But in many church buildings, you'll have more privacy and fewer comments from passersby if you nurse in a pew during the worship service rather than in the women's rest room or even the nursery. If you breastfeed the baby before he starts to cry, most people won't know what you're doing.

- Many public places are providing areas especially for mothers to nurse their babies. Look for these; use them; and if you get a chance, write a note of appreciation. But don't feel that you have to hide in a special nursing mothers' facility when you visit that major theme park. It's often much more convenient just to breastfeed wherever you can.

What to Do If Someone Complains

Many states have passed special laws affirming a woman's right to breastfeed her baby in public places without fear of someone citing local ordinances about indecent exposure. There's also a federal law to this effect about breastfeeding on federal property. While occasionally mothers breastfeeding in restaurants, stores, or at the public pool have sparked local controversies, no one has ever gotten into trouble with the law for breastfeeding in a public place. Breastfeeding in public never has been against the law. Fortunately, public opinion on breastfeeding is becoming more enlightened as the benefits of breastfeeding become more widely recognized. While stories about women being asked not to nurse in restaurants occasionally make headlines, in the brouhaha that follows, most commentators come down squarely on the side of the nursing mother. It's good public relations for businesses and public facilities to accommodate the needs of breastfeeding families.

Thousands and thousands of mothers in the U.S. nurse their babies every day at the mall, the park, or the pool and other people either don't notice, don't care, or smile approvingly. Millions more mothers around the world think nothing of nursing wherever they may be. Chances are, no one will ever hassle you about nursing in public (at least no strangers—friends and family are another issue). If someone does express disapproval, be polite, be firm—but there's no need to run and hide or even apologize. This is the 21st century after all, and you're giving your baby the most technologically advanced nutrition available!

How to Help Others Feel More Comfortable

For some mothers, the biggest obstacle to nursing in public is their own mind set: "Nursing in public may be fine for someone else, but it's just not me." You may not feel instantly comfortable nursing your baby anywhere and everywhere, but start small and give it a try. Once you've experienced the freedom of being able to grab a few diapers and go, you may decide that when it comes to convenience, breastfeeding is the original fast food.

Sometimes people who are not accustomed to being around nursing babies simply don't know where to look while baby has his dinner. You can help them out by maintaining eye contact with this other person while your baby is latching on. That will help observers focus on your face and avoid looking at your breast, which will probably help them feel more comfortable. A brief positive comment about your breastfed baby will also help people who are new to the world of babies feel more at ease.

Many mothers find it easier to nurse around strangers than around certain friends or members of their extended family. What do you do if your father-in-law leaves the living room while you nurse? Or if your husband doesn't want you nursing your baby in front of his softball buddies? A lot depends on the relationships, but in many cases it just takes time for people who are unfamiliar with breastfeeding to feel comfortable about it. Eventually, people who care about you and your baby will take their cue from you. If you're comfortable nursing in front of the television during the World Series, surrounded by friends old and new, these friends will soon learn to be comfortable too.

When you first venture out into public with your baby, bring along a friend. A more experienced nursing mother can supply the confidence you need. So can a supportive husband. And smile proudly—you're doing the best for your baby.

About the Author

Dr. William Sears, M.D. is Associate Clinical Professor of Pediatrics at the University of California, Irvine, School of Medicine, and the co-author of numerous books on childbirth and parenting including *The Baby Book* (Little Brown & Co., 1992) and *The Breastfeeding Book* (Little Brown & Co., 2000). He is also a medical and parenting consultant for *BabyTalk* and *Parenting* magazines. Additional information about Dr. Sears can be found at www.askdrsears.com/aboutdrsears.asp.

Chapter 26

Breastfeeding and International Travel

When deciding to travel, a pregnant woman should be advised to consider the potential problems associated with international travel, as well as the quality of medical care available at her destination and during transit. The decision to travel internationally while nursing produces its own challenges. However, breastfeeding has nutritional and anti-infective advantages that serve an infant well while traveling. Therefore, breastfeeding should be advised. Moreover, exclusive breastfeeding relieves concerns about sterilizing bottles and about availability of clean water. Supplements are usually not needed by breastfed infants younger than 6 months of age, and breastfeeding should be maintained as long as possible. If supplementation is considered necessary, powdered formula that requires reconstitution with boiled water should be carried. For short trips, it may be feasible to carry an adequate supply of pre-prepared canned formula.

Nursing women may be immunized for maximum protection, depending on the travel itinerary. However, consideration needs to be given to the neonate who cannot be immunized at birth and who would not gain protection against many infections (for example, yellow fever, measles, and meningococcal meningitis) through breastfeeding.

Neither inactivated nor live virus vaccines affect the safety of breastfeeding for mothers or infants. Breastfeeding does not adversely affect immunization and is not a contraindication to the administration

Excerpted from "Pregnancy, Breastfeeding, and Travel: Health Information for International Travel, 1999–2000," last reviewed July 2000. Centers for Disease Control and Prevention, www.cdc.gov.

of any vaccines, including live virus vaccines, for breastfeeding women. Although rubella vaccine virus may be transmitted in breastmilk, the virus usually does not infect the infant; if it does, the infection is well tolerated. Breastfed infants should be vaccinated according to routine recommended schedules.

Nursing women should be advised that their eating and sleeping patterns, as well as stress, will inevitably affect their milk output. They need to increase their fluid intake; avoid excess alcohol and caffeine; and, as much as possible, avoid exposure to tobacco smoke.

Breastfeeding is desirable during travel and should be continued as long as possible because of its safety and the resulting lower incidence of infant diarrhea. A nursing mother with travelers' diarrhea should not stop breastfeeding, but should increase her fluid intake.

Women traveling with neonates or infants should be advised to check with their pediatricians regarding any medical contraindications to flying. Infants are particularly susceptible to pain with Eustachian tube collapse during pressure changes. Breastfeeding during ascent and descent relieves this discomfort.

Additions and substitutions to the usual travel health kit need to be made during pregnancy and nursing. Talcum powder, a thermometer, oral rehydration salt (ORS) packets, multivitamins, an antifungal agent for vaginal yeast, acetaminophen, insect repellent containing a low percentage of DEET (diethyltoluamide), and a sunscreen with a high SPF (sun protection factor) should be carried. Antimalarial and antidiarrheal self-treatment medications should be evaluated individually depending on the traveler, the itinerary, and her health history. Most medications should be avoided, if possible.

Chapter 27

How to Wean Your Baby

Deciding to Wean

Are you really ready to wean completely? Sometimes just cutting back on the amount of times you breastfeed will make you feel better. Breastfeeding is a two-way street. If you resent it most times you sit down to breastfeed, your child will pick up on this. If your baby is under a year (or older, sometimes), you will have to substitute a bottle feeding for a missed breastfeeding. An older baby may accept a drink from a cup, a nutritious snack, or just a distraction in the form of a game, a toy, or change of scene. Remember, the first supplemental feed—from a bottle or of solid food—is the beginning of weaning.

If weaning is your decision, it's best for you and your baby to do it gradually, and with love. If you wean "cold turkey," your breasts will likely become painfully engorged, and you might develop a breast infection. Your baby will probably fight the switch from your warm, soft breast to a plastic substitute. He might mourn the loss of "his" breasts.

Weaning an Infant

To wean a baby under a year, substitute his least favorite feeding first. If the baby won't accept the bottle from you, see if Daddy or Grandma can succeed. Let the baby have a few days (or weeks, if pos-

---

"FAQ on How to Wean," last updated 1999. ©1999 La Leche League International (LLLI), www.laleleague.org. Reprinted with permission.

sible) between each time you substitute a breastfeeding session with a bottle. Express a little milk from your breasts, for your own comfort, if you become engorged. Don't express a whole feeding's worth of milk; just take the pressure off. Your body will get the signal to make less milk over time.

Weaning an Older Baby

Do you want to wean a baby who is a year or older? You may not need to go to bottles at all. All you may need to do is stop offering the breast. "Don't offer, don't refuse" may work for you. Substitute solid food or a cup of water, juice, or cow's milk (if tolerated) for the least important feeding. Sometimes Dad (or another relative) can help by taking the baby to the kitchen for a good breakfast. This can become a special time for both of them, and you get some extra sleep! For mealtime feeds, try to offer food first, with a short session at the breast for later. Avoid sitting down in your special favorite nursing chair. If your child won't nap without breastfeeding, sometimes a car ride will get him or her to sleep.

The nighttime feeding is usually the last to go. Make a bedtime routine not centered around breastfeeding. A good book or two will eventually become more important than a long session at the breast. Your child may agree to rest his head on your breast instead of feeding. Talk to your child about what's going on. He may understand more than you think.

A lot of extra love and attention in other forms will be needed now. Try getting out more to the playground, a friend's house, shopping, museums, or anywhere your child will be distracted by. Read stories, rub or scratch their little back, or sing and dance. It's a whole new stage in your growing child's life. You will still be needed, just in different ways.

Chapter 28

Nutrition for the Nursing Mother

Breastfeeding your infant doesn't require a complicated set of diet rules. However, taking care of your nutritional health can help you feel better, both physically and psychologically.

Nutrition Recommendations for Nursing Mothers

Avoid Crash Dieting or Rapid Weight Loss

During the first six months of exclusive breastfeeding, breastmilk contains about 650 calories per day. Following the recommendations to consume 500 calories more each day than you did before becoming pregnant means you'll experience a gradual weight loss of about one and one-half to two pounds per month (based on the USDA Food Guide Pyramid and a 2700 calorie per day diet).

Eat a Balanced Diet

Fruits and vegetables are particularly important because they contain needed folate and magnesium, while meats and poultry provide for your increased vitamin B6, iron, and zinc needs. Also, don't forget your calcium. The USDA's Food Guide Pyramid can help you get all these important nutrients every day.

From "Nursing Nutrition," USDA/ARS Children's Nutrition Research Center at Baylor College of Medicine. ©1999 Baylor College of Medicine, used with permission.

Eat a Variety of Foods

A healthy diet includes many different foods. A variety of aromas and flavors in breastmilk are thought to enhance weaning to solid foods. However, should your infant appear sensitive to certain foods you eat, keep a record and eliminate those that consistently cause problems.

Drink Plenty of Liquids

If you rarely feel thirsty, check your urine. Dark yellow urine is a sure sign that your fluid intake is low.

Use Caffeine in Moderation

If your infant is fussy or irritable, caffeine could be the culprit. Newborns are particularly sensitive to caffeine and alcohol.

Use Alcohol in Moderation, If at All

If you choose to drink alcohol, moderation is the key. Limit yourself to one or two small drinks on special occasions and wait two to four hours before breastfeeding to allow your milk to be cleared of alcohol.

Table 28.1. Daily Dietary Guidelines for Breastfeeding Mothers

Food Group	Number of Servings	Serving Size
Grain	10	1 slice of bread, ½ c. cooked rice, cereal or pasta
Fruit	4	¾ c. juice, 1 med. piece of fresh fruit, ½ c. canned fruit
Vegetable	5	½ c. chopped, 1 c. leafy green, ¾ c. juice
Dairy	3–4	1 c. milk or yogurt, 1 ½ ounce cheese
Meat	6	1 oz. = ½ c. beans, 1 egg, 2 T. peanut butter

Note: In the sample diet shown in Table 28.1, the daily total fat intake is 90 grams, 30 grams of which are saturated fat. There are 17 teaspoons of added sugar (one teaspoon is four grams). Nursing mothers over 18 years of age need 3 servings per day from the dairy group, while those 18 years and younger need 4 servings.

Consult Your Physician

Check with your physician before taking any over-the-counter vitamins, nutritional or herbal supplements, or medications.

Nutritional Guidelines for Nursing Mothers

Although individual needs vary, the energy RDA set by the Food and Nutrition Board of the National Academy of Sciences for average-size, normally active women is 2200 calories per day. This means that most nursing moms need about 2700 calories per day.

Chapter 29

Is It Safe to Lose Weight While Breastfeeding?

A study by National Institute of Child Health and Human Development (NICHD)-funded researchers has found that overweight mothers who breastfeed their infants may lose weight through a sensible diet and exercise program without fear of harming their infants. The study, appearing in the February 17, 2000 *New England Journal of Medicine*, was conducted by Cheryl A. Lovelady, Ph.D. and her coworkers at the University of North Carolina in Greensboro.

"Being overweight may cause serious health problems," said NICHD Director Duane Alexander, M.D. "This study shows that it's safe for overweight women to begin a sensible weight loss program without posing a risk to their infants."

Dr. Lovelady explained that weight gained during pregnancy might contribute to obesity later in life. Losing this extra weight soon after pregnancy may help many women to avoid later obesity and its long-term health effects. An Institute of Medicine report earlier had concluded that overweight breastfeeding women could probably lose about two kg (4.4 pounds) per month without affecting their production of milk. However, Dr. Lovelady pointed out, no studies existed to prove whether this assumption was true.

Dr. Lovelady stressed that a woman who is breastfeeding should first consult her physician and nutritionist before undertaking any

From "Moderate Weight Loss OK for Overweight Moms Who Breast Feed," February 2000, News Release. National Institute of Child Health and Human Development (NICHD), www.nichd.nih.gov.

weight loss program. She added that breastfeeding women should not attempt to lose weight if they are only a few pounds overweight.

"Breastfeeding mothers who are only 5 pounds overweight shouldn't try to lose weight," she said. Unless a woman has sufficient fat reserves, dieting may hinder milk production and also cause the woman to feel fatigued.

The researchers recruited forty overweight, breastfeeding women for the study. The women took part in the study for ten weeks, beginning at the fourth week after they gave birth. Overweight was defined as having a body mass index of 25 to 30. Body mass index is a mathematical formula used to calculate body fat from a person's height and weight. Dr. Lovelady explained that a 5' 4" woman having a body mass index of from 25 to 30 would weigh between 145 and 175 pounds. The authors wrote that 51 percent of U.S. women have a body mass index of more than 25.

Of the forty women, twenty-one were assigned to the diet and exercise group, and nineteen were assigned to the control group. All the women had given birth to full-term, full-size infants delivered without C-section. Women in the diet and exercise group reduced their food intake by 500 calories, essentially by avoiding fatty and sugary foods. These women also began some form of aerobic exercise such as brisk walking, jogging, or aerobic dancing for fifteen minutes a day. The exercise time was increased by two minutes a day, until the women were exercising for forty-five minutes a day. To help the women stick to their diets, the researchers also provided them with six low-fat, low-sugar frozen entrees per week during the course of the study.

The control group exercised no more than once a week, and did not change their dietary habits. All the women received a daily multivitamin containing at least 50 percent of the recommended daily allowances for breastfeeding women.

The women in the diet and exercise group lost an average of about 5 kilograms (about ten pounds) by the end of ten weeks. The women in the control group lost an average of .8 kilograms (about two pounds). In contrast to the diet-and-exercise group, which lost weight at about the same rate, the control group varied in their weight loss. In fact, a few of the women lost nearly ten pounds, while a few others gained that amount.

The women in the diet-and-exercise group reported that they seemed to be producing enough milk. Also, they reported that their infants were not crying any more than normal. (Infant fussiness is a possible indication of insufficient milk production.) Similarly, the women did not report feeling tired. In fact, most said that the exercise sessions seemed to give them more energy.

The infants of the women in the diet and exercise group grew at a normal rate, as compared both to the infants of the women in the control group as well as to those in larger studies of infant growth.

"In conclusion," the authors wrote, "a program of moderate exercise and energy restriction was successful in inducing weight loss in overweight, lactating mothers without harming the growth of their infants in the early postpartum period."

The study builds upon the findings of an earlier study, published in the *New England Journal of Medicine* on February 17, 1994. This study found that breastfeeding mothers could not lose weight if they began an exercise program without also cutting the amount of calories they consumed. "You've got to have the caloric restriction if you're going to see weight loss," Dr. Lovelady said.

Chapter 30

Fathers and Breastfeeding

Feelings of jealousy and of being left out are a normal reaction in some fathers to the intimate relationship between a nursing mother and her baby. The best way to avoid these kinds of feelings is to be an active participant in your new baby's life and the way he or she is fed. The following are just some of the ways a new father can be involved in the care and feeding of his breastfed infant.

As a New Father You Can

- Bring the baby to the mother when it's time to nurse.
- Change the baby's diaper before or after nursings.
- Hold the baby while mother gets herself into a comfortable nursing position.
- Help to rouse the baby if she's too sleepy to nurse.
- Get your partner something to drink while she is nursing. Nursing mothers are always thirsty and need extra fluids.
- Take over the child care between nursings so the mother can get some rest or time to herself.
- Do grocery shopping and keep nutritious snacks on hand.

University of Rhode Island Cooperative Extension Expanded Food and Nutrition Program (EFNEP), www.uri.edu, undated. Reprinted with permission of the University of Rhode Island.

- Share in the household chores.

- Reassure your partner that she is doing a good job and that you think what she is doing is important.

If Problems Arise

Difficulties which arise in the early weeks of breastfeeding can seem overwhelming to the mother who is exhausted from lack of sleep or experiencing pain. Some women question their ability to continue nursing during this time. It is at this point that the support and encouragement of the father can contribute greatly to the success of breastfeeding. You can help offset common concerns and problems.

Doubts about Having Enough Milk

This is a real concern for many women. REASSURE your partner that the baby is getting plenty of milk if:

- The baby nurses eight to twelve times in twenty-four hours.

- The baby has at least six wet and two dirty diapers in twenty-four hours.

- The baby gains four to seven ounces per week.

- The baby is content between feedings.

Breastfeeding works by supply and demand. The more often the infant is put to the breast, the more milk the mother will have.

Sore Nipples

This problem is most often caused by poor positioning of the baby to the breast. With your partner, check that your baby is latching onto the areola (brown part) of the breast and not just sucking on the nipple itself. Remind mom to alternate nursing positions and to air dry her nipples for ten to twenty minutes after each feeding.

Chapter 31

Birth Control Options

Deciding what method of birth control to use is not easy. Your health care provider will encourage you to make a decision about a birth control method around the 27th to 28th week of your pregnancy. This will give you time to make a good decision for yourself.

Remember, you can get pregnant right after delivery of your baby even if you do not have a period.

Some questions to ask yourself:

1. Do I have any medical problems that may affect my choice of birth control methods?

2. Which birth control option is going to be most effective for me? What will I do if the method fails?

3. Which type of birth control is easiest for me to use?

4. How much does my choice of birth control cost?

5. Does my partner support my decision?

6. Do I need a method to protect me against sexually transmitted diseases and HIV?

7. Will the birth control choice affect my milk supply if I choose to breastfeed?

8. Do I want more children in the future?

From the University of Iowa Healthbook (Virtual Hospital), www.vh.org. Last revised July 2000; reprinted with permission.

Table 31.1. Choosing the Right Birth Control

Method: Abstinence

Reliability: 100%

What Is It and How Does It Work? You don't get pregnant if you don't have sex.

Advantages: You are protected from sexually transmitted disease and HIV.

Drawbacks: Most people do not wish to abstain from sex.

Method: Norplant

Reliability: 99% or more.

What Is It and How Does It Work? Six flexible capsules of hormones, about the size of a match stick, placed under the skin surface of your arm by a doctor. Hormones released thicken the cervical mucus and prevent sperm from getting to the egg. May also prevent the release of the egg from the ovaries.

Advantages: Very effective and simple to use. Lasts for 5 years and works well for those wanting this time before another possible pregnancy. Is removed by a health care provider. Safe for breastfeeding mothers.

Drawbacks: Minor surgery for placement and removal. Payment for the method is all at the time of placement of the capsules. Thus, the initial cost is high but the method lasts for five years. May cause some changes in periods with spotting and missed periods. No protection against sexually transmitted disease and HIV. Possible side effects include weight gain, headaches, or mood changes.

Method: Depo-Provera (DMPA)

Reliability: 99% or more.

What Is It and How Does It Work? A shot (hormone) is given every three months to prevent the ovaries from releasing an egg. Also, changes the lining of the uterus (womb). Will need to use another birth control method the first two weeks for protection against pregnancy. Must get from a health care provider.

Advantages: Safe and effective and simple to use. Usually have no menstrual periods while getting the injections. Safe for breastfeeding mothers.

Table 31.1. Choosing the Right Birth Control, continued.

Method: **Depo-Provera (DMPA), continued**

Drawbacks: Commonly causes irregular bleeding. Possible side effects include weight gain, headaches, or mood changes. No protection against sexually transmitted disease and HIV.

Method: **Oral Birth Control Pills**

Reliability: 97–99% if you never miss a pill.

What Is It and How Does It Work? Hormones that are taken by mouth each day that stop the ovaries from releasing an egg. Must get prescription from a health care provider.

Advantages: Very effective, safe, and simple to use. Progestin-only (mini-pill) is suggested for breastfeeding mothers as it is less likely to affect milk supply. May want to use a different method of birth control until breastfeeding is well established (generally around six to eight weeks after delivery).

Drawbacks: Pill must be taken at about the same time every day to be effective against pregnancy. Possible side effects include weight gain, headaches, and mood changes. No protection against sexually transmitted diseases and HIV.

Method: **IUD**

Reliability: 97%

What Is It and How Does It Work? Health care provider inserts a small thin, flexible T-shaped device inside the uterus (womb) to prevent pregnancy. A small string attached to the device protrudes from the cervix and the woman can feel the string inside her vagina. This is to ensure the device is in place.

Advantages: Safe, effective, and simple to use. Effective for eight or more years. Can be removed by a health care provider whenever you want to become pregnant.

Drawbacks: May cause increased cramping during periods. Not a good choice for women at risk for sexually transmitted diseases. Does not protect against (and may promote development of problems related to) sexually transmitted diseases and HIV.

Table 31.1. Choosing the Right Birth Control, continued.

Method: Condom

Reliability: 88% and up to 96% if used correctly every time with foam.

What Is It and How Does It Work? Latex or rubber covering which fits tightly over the penis. Collects the sperm and semen. Most reliable if the woman also uses spermicidal foam, jelly, or creams.

Advantages: Must be placed on an erect penis and removed after climax. Can buy in most drugstores and is inexpensive. Can only be used once and thrown away.

Drawbacks: Must be put on immediately before lovemaking. Can tear easily with rough handling. Can dull man's sexual feeling. Irritation of the penis may happen when used with spermicidal foams, jellies, or creams. Can offer protection from sexually transmitted diseases and HIV.

Method: Diaphragm or Cervical Cap

Reliability: 82% and up to 94% if carefully used each time.

What Is It and How Does It Work? Small rubber cup fits inside vagina and over the cervix (opening) of the uterus (womb). Best to use with spermicides. Must be fitted by a health care provider.

Advantages: Can be put into place two hours before lovemaking. Use only during intercourse.

Drawbacks: Can be messy and needs to remain in place for six to eight hours after intercourse. Use of foam, jellies, and creams may cause irritation to the vagina and cervix.

Method: Rhythm (Natural Family Planning)

Reliability: 80%

What Is It and How Does It Work? Woman looks for body signs each day to check for fertile periods: cervical mucus, body temperature, and day of cycle. Women need to chart the signs for a few months to make more accurate predictions of fertile and non fertile times.

Advantages: No medication. Acceptable for most religious groups. Calendar, thermometer, and chart are easy to get.

Drawbacks: Takes time and practice to understand the meaning of daily charting. Protection against pregnancy occurs by avoiding fertile times. Does not protect against sexually transmitted diseases and HIV.

Table 31.1 lists the most common types of birth control. Feel free to talk to your health care provider about any concerns or questions you may have.

Many breastfeeding mothers are interested in how well breastfeeding works as a birth control method. Breastfeeding is effective in preventing ovulation and possible pregnancy if you do not supplement with formula at all. This means the baby receives no liquids, no solids other than mother's milk—day and night, and no pacifiers. For best protection, an additional type of birth control is recommended.

Part Five

Breastfeeding Difficulties

Chapter 32

Breast and Nipple Soreness: Causes, Prevention, and Treatment

Chapter Contents

Section 32.1

Identifying the Problem

From "Sore Breasts," at www.askdrsears.com, undated, by Dr. William P.
Sears © AskDrSears.com. Used with permission. Information about Dr. Sears
can be found at the end of this chapter or at www.askdrsears.com.

Pain in the breasts may be caused by engorgement, a plugged duct, mastitis, or something else. It is often difficult for a mother (and doctor) to tell whether the inflammation is due to engorgement or a plugged duct (neither of which needs antibiotics) or mastitis (which usually, but not always, requires antibiotics). Use the guidelines in Table 32.1 to help you figure out what the problem is and how to treat it. Find additional information on how to relieve sore breasts in the following sections of this chapter.

Table 32.1. Sore Breasts: Stages of Severity

Features	Normal Breast Fullness	Engorge-ment	Plugged Duct	Mastitis
Usual onset:	2–4 days after birth	Within the first two weeks	Most noticeable after feed-ings	Most common around third week postpar-tum; may occur at any time dur-ing lactating.
Location:	Both breasts	Both breasts	Localized area in one breast	One breast
Breasts feel:	Generally swollen, uncomfortable, not hard, but tight	Hard, swollen, sore, warm	Mildly tender lump beneath areola, red-dened skin above	Very painful: hot, tender, swollen, red streaking
Maternal fever:	None	101°F or below	None	Higher than 101°F
Mother generally feels:	Well	Well	Well; may see a white milk plug in a nipple opening.	Achy, tired, chills, flu-like symptoms
Treatment:	Frequent, unrestricted feeding; empty breasts	Frequent, unrestricted feeding; empty breasts, alter-nating warm and cold com-presses, rest	Frequent, unrestricted feeding; moist, hot packs; massage plugged duct to loosen plug and encourage milk flow	Frequent, unrestricted feeding; empty breasts; rest and relaxation; physician may prescribe antibiotics

Section 32.2

Engorgement

"Engorgement" from www.askdrsears.com, undated, by Dr. William P.
Sears © AskDrSears.com. Used with permission. Information about Dr. Sears
can be found at the end of this chapter or at www.askdrsears.com.

Two to four days after birth, mothers may awaken to find their
breasts have grown two cup sizes overnight. It's those milk-making
hormones at work! "Has your milk come in yet?" asks the nurse. Mom
can answer with a definite "yes!"

This dramatic increase in breast size and fullness is called physiologic engorgement. It is caused by postpartum changes in hormone
levels, which kick off the milk production process and also increase
blood circulation to the breasts.

It's not that you didn't have milk before. Your body began producing colostrum, the first milk, late in pregnancy and made more immediately after birth as your newborn feeds at your breast. It's more
accurate to say that the milk supply suddenly increases rather than
to say it "comes in." Physiologic engorgement is usually more dramatic
and uncomfortable in first-time mothers and lessens in intensity with
subsequent pregnancies.

The sudden fullness and tightness may be a bit uncomfortable
during those early days when your breasts seem to fill up faster than
your baby can empty them. Some mothers even run a slight fever
when their breasts are engorged.

Frequent breastfeeding is the best way to prevent and treat engorgement. Relief comes when baby gets the milk flowing and empties the
breast. Once you and your baby settle into a comfortable balance of
milk production where the supply equals the demand, the discomfort
will pass. The swelling will subside and your breasts won't be so enormous, but they will continue to make milk steadily and efficiently.

Preventing and Coping with Engorgement

Engorgement can lead to other problems, so it's important to treat
it promptly. When the breasts swell with fluid and milk, the nipple

may flatten out, making it more difficult for baby to latch on correctly. Baby can suck on only the end of the nipple and can't get enough of the areolar tissue into her mouth to compress the milk sinuses and empty the breast. Engorgement gets worse, while baby remains hungry. As the hungry baby sucks harder but incorrectly, the nipple gets traumatized and painfully sore. Eventually, the body decides not to make so much milk, which ends the engorgement, but may lead to problems with milk supply if baby is still not latching on and sucking well. Fortunately, you can keep normal physiologic engorgement from becoming a problem. Here are some suggestions for coping with breast fullness:

- Teach baby efficient latch-on in the first days after birth. It's easier for a baby to learn to latch on correctly on the first and second day when your breasts are softer, before your milk comes in. Baby should grasp the breast with a wide-open mouth.

- Room-in with your baby immediately after birth and breastfeed frequently. This will minimize problems with engorgement and get your milk supply attuned to baby's needs more quickly.

- Nurse often during the night as well as during the day. In the first month or two, a baby who sleeps for four or five hours at a time is a mixed blessing. Mother gets a chance to rest, but her breasts become engorged. Wake baby every two hours during the day and don't let him sleep for more than four hours at night.

- Do not limit the length of feedings to five or ten minutes to protect your nipples. Protect your nipples by being sure that baby latches on correctly. Limiting the length of feedings will increase engorgement because in the beginning, baby can not adequately empty the breasts in five or ten minutes.

- Use a hospital-grade electric breast pump to release some of the milk if you are becoming uncomfortably engorged and baby is not nursing well or often enough. This will soften the areola and allow baby to latch on more efficiently and thus empty your breasts. Or gently use hand expression to release some milk. Express only enough milk to make you feel more comfortable. Expressing too much milk may stimulate the production of more milk. Remember, the production of milk works on the supply and demand principle.

- Soak your breasts in a warm shower just before expressing your milk or feeding your baby. Direct the shower spray from the top of your breast toward your nipple as you massage your breasts. This warmth helps trigger your milk ejection reflex, which gets the milk flowing more quickly when you begin to pump or baby begins to feed. Other ways to apply warmth and moisture to your breasts include leaning over a basin of warm water (gravity will help you express milk in this position) or applying warm compresses to your breasts.

- If baby is unable to nurse well, you need to pump your milk with an electric pump every 2 to 3 hours to prevent problems with engorgement and to keep your milk production up. Basically, do whatever you need to do to get your milk out of your breasts. Frequent emptying of the breasts in the early stages of lactation will help you have a good milk supply in the weeks and months to come.

- Above all, don't stop breastfeeding. Unrelieved engorgement can lead to a breast infection, and a baby who nurses well can empty the breasts more efficiently than any pump.

- Between feedings, apply cold compresses to your breasts to relieve the pain and reduce swelling. Wrap small plastic bags filled with crushed ice in a lightweight dishtowel. Crushed ice is less heavy on tender breasts, or try bags of frozen vegetables.

- Wear a loose fitting bra. Avoid bras that are too tight and/or that compress the lower part of your breast against your body. This traps milk and sets you up for engorgement and possible mastitis.

- Rest, rest, rest! Lie down with your baby and nurse and nap together. There's something magical about the way rest relieves engorgement.

- What about using cabbage leaves to treat engorgement? So far, controlled studies have shown no benefit to this treatment over the standard treatments listed above. Yet some mothers find this works very well, and it's easier than trying to balance ice packs on your chest. Use clean cabbage leaves. Make a hole for the nipple and tuck them into your bra for twenty to thirty minutes. Repeat two or three times a day until engorgement is relieved.

Engorgement after the Early Weeks

If you have enjoyed weeks of trouble-free breastfeeding and then suddenly become engorged, take this as a signal that something is interfering with the balance between your milk supply and baby's demand. Your baby is going too long between feedings, isn't nursing well, or stress is affecting your nursing pattern or your milk-ejection reflex. Veteran breastfeeding mothers take engorgement as a cue to take a few days off from other responsibilities to reconnect with baby. They increase the frequency and duration of feedings and soon resettle into a comfortable breastfeeding pattern.

Section 32.3

Plugged Ducts

From "Plugged Milk Ducts," at www.askdrsears.com, undated, by Dr. William P. Sears © AskDrSears.com. Used with permission. Information about Dr. Sears can be found at the end of this chapter or at www.askdrsears.com.

Sometimes a milk duct leading from the milk-making cells to the nipple gets plugged, resulting in a tender lump beneath the areola. There may also be a wedge-shaped area of redness extending from the lump back towards the wall of the chest. Unlike mastitis, the pain comes and goes with a plugged duct, and unless the duct is infected you will not feel generally ill. If left untreated, however, a plugged duct may become infected, resulting in mastitis, infection, or a breast abscess.

To unplug the duct and prevent subsequent infection, try these suggestions:

- Continue to breastfeed on the affected side. By any means, get the milk out! This is the golden rule of preventing engorgement, plugged ducts, and mastitis. Use a breast pump or hand expression if baby is unwilling to nurse.

- Breastfeed on the affected side first. Baby's sucking is strongest at the beginning of the feed, so he is more likely to dislodge the plug when he starts on the affected breast.

- Vary the baby's position at the breast, so that all of the milk ducts are drained. Be sure the baby is latched on well, so that he can nurse efficiently. Try the clutch hold or side-lying position. Before each feeding, massage the affected area by kneading your breast gently from the top of the breast down over the plugged duct toward the nipple.

- Drain the affected breast better by positioning baby so his chin "points" to the area that is sore. For example, if the lump is around 4 o'clock, use the clutch hold and position baby's chin around this point on the nipple clock. The lower jaw is often most effective at getting milk out of the breast.

- Apply moist heat compresses for a few minutes before feeding or pumping, or soak the affected breast in warm water or in the shower.

- Rest. Lie down with the baby and nap while you nurse.

- If you notice a small white dot at the end of the milk duct on your nipple, that is the end of a plugged nipple opening. Apply moist heat on this white blister and with a sterile needle gently pop the blister. If this pore stays plugged, it could block milk drainage and lead to a plugged duct and mastitis.

- Try a pressure massage on the area of your breast that is swollen and painful because of a plugged duct. This may help to loosen the plug. With pressure massage, you do not actually move your hand over the skin as you would with a normal massage. You simply press more and more firmly with the heel of your hand to move the plug in the duct down closer to the nipple, as described below.

To do pressure massage, start at the edge of the lumpy area closest to your chest wall. Apply pressure to that area with the heel of your hand to the point just before it becomes too painful. Hold the pressure at that level until the pain eases off. Then increase the pressure again, without moving your hand, and hold it until the pain eases. Continue to gradually increase pressure at that same site until you are pressing as hard as you can. Then pick your hand up, move it down toward your nipple about a half inch, and repeat the pressure massage in this area. Continue moving your hand a half inch and repeating the massage until you get all the way down to the nipple.

You may see the dried milk come out from an opening in your nipple. Even if the plug doesn't actually come out, you will at least have dislodged it and moved it toward the nipple so that when baby goes to the breast and sucks, he will remove it with his suction. Always put baby to the breast on the plugged side first, when his sucking will be the strongest.

Preventing Plugged Ducts from Recurring

- To prevent plugged ducts, feed baby in different positions with his nose pointing "around the nipple clock," so that you empty all the milk sinuses and ducts.

- Studies have shown that taking a tablespoon a day of oral granular lecithin or a capsule of 1,200 mg lecithin capsule three to four times a day is helpful in preventing and treating plugged milk ducts.

Section 32.4

Mastitis

"Mastitis," from www.askdrsears.com, undated, by Dr. William P. Sears © AskDrSears.com. Used with permission. Information about Dr. Sears can be found at the end of this chapter or at www.askdrsears.com.

Mastitis means that the breast is inflamed and there is swelling, redness, tenderness, and pain. There may be an infection, so it is wise to consult your health-care provider to determine whether or not an antibiotic is necessary. A breast infection can become a breast abscess that requires surgical draining, but this can almost always be prevented by treating mastitis promptly.

The following signs indicate that you might have mastitis.

- Part or all of the breast is intensely painful, hot, tender, red, and swollen. Some mothers can pinpoint a definite area of inflammation, while at other times the entire breast is tender.

161

- If you feel tired, run down, or achy; or if you have chills, feel feverish, or have a temperature 101°F or higher then your symptoms suggest that you have an infection A breastfeeding mother who thinks she has the flu probably has mastitis. Mothers with mastitis will sometimes experience these flu-like symptoms even before they get a fever or notice breast tenderness.

- You are feeling progressively worse, your breasts are growing more tender, and your fever is becoming more pronounced. With simple engorgement, a plugged duct, or mastitis without infection, you gradually feel better instead of worse.

- Recent events have set you up for mastitis: cracked or bleeding nipples, stress or getting run down, missed feedings, or longer intervals between feedings.

Preventing Mastitis

The best way to prevent mastitis is to avoid the situations that set you up for it.

- Relieve engorgement promptly. Milk that doesn't flow gets thicker and clogs the ducts, which is a set up for mastitis.

- Breastfeed frequently. Don't restrict the length of feedings.

- Encourage your baby to nurse. You don't have to wait for baby to tell you he's hungry if you feel your breasts getting full.

- Sleep wisely. Avoid sleeping on your stomach or so far over on your side that your breasts are compressed against the mattress.

- Take care of yourself. Get plenty of rest for your mind and body.

Problems with recurrent mastitis are usually the result of irregular breastfeeding patterns like missing feedings, giving bottles in place of breastfeedings, or skipping pumping sessions when separated from the baby. Recurrent mastitis may also mean that mother's immune system is generally run down because of fatigue and stress. Mastitis is a sign that you need to take a closer look at your lifestyle and breastfeeding relationship and make some adjustments.

Treating Mastitis

Treating mastitis is much like treating engorgement only more urgent. Follow the suggestions for treating engorgement in Section 32.2, as well as the following:

- Rest, rest, rest. Mastitis is an illness, so take a medical leave from all responsibilities other than breastfeeding. Take your baby to bed with you and nurse. Rest relieves stress and replenishes your immune system.

- Alternate warm and cold compresses on your breasts. Cold compresses relieve pain, and warmth increases circulation, which mobilizes infection fighters in the inflamed area. Lean over a basin of warm water, stand in a warm shower, or soak in a warm bath. Warm water or a warm, wet towel is more effective than the dry heat of a heating pad. For cold compresses, use crushed ice in plastic bags or bags of frozen vegetables, covered with a thin dishtowel to protect your skin.

- Gently massage the area of tenderness. This increases circulation, helps to loosen any plugged ducts in the area, and mobilizes local immune factors. Try doing this while soaking the breast in a warm shower or bath.

- Breastfeed frequently on the affected side. If it hurts to nurse the baby, start the feeding on the breast that is not sore and switch to the sore side after your milk lets down. Breastfeeding is usually more comfortable when the milk is flowing. It's important to empty the inflamed breast. As in other parts of the body, fluid that is trapped can get infected. Your baby can empty your breast more efficiently than a breast pump. However, if your baby is not nursing well, you may have to use a breast pump or hand expression to get the milk out.

- Vary the baby's position at the breast so that all the ducts are emptied.

- Take analgesics for fever and pain. Acetaminophen and/or ibuprofen are safe to take while breastfeeding. Unrelieved pain not only decreases your ability to produce milk, but suppresses your body's ability to fight infection.

- Drink lots of fluids, like you would if you had the flu. Fever and inflammation increase your need for fluids.

- Boost your immune system with good nutrition.

- Sleep without a bra. At other times, wear a looser-fitting bra that does not put pressure on the affected area. If possible, go without a bra.

- Don't quit nursing at this point. Weaning increases the risk of a breast infection turning into a breast abscess that requires surgical draining. Continuing to nurse your baby is the best treatment for engorgement, mastitis, and breast infections.

- If baby refuses to nurse on the affected breast, it may be because inflammation of the milk glands increases the sodium content of your milk, giving it a salty taste. Most babies either don't notice or don't mind, and go right on nursing. Some may object to the change and fuss or refuse to nurse from that side. Try starting the feeding on the unaffected side and finishing on the salty side. As the inflammation subsides, your milk will soon return to its usual taste.

Do You Need Antibiotic Treatment?

You can experience the pain and inflammation of mastitis without necessarily having a bacterial infection. Yet it is often difficult to tell whether mastitis has become a breast infection. Consult your health care provider as soon as you suspect mastitis. In our medical practice, we operate on the principle of better to treat mastitis earlier than later. Mothers who are given antibiotics too late in the course of mastitis are more likely to wean their babies from the breast, to have a more severe infection, and to have the infection recur.

The following guidelines can help you both determine whether or not you need an antibiotic.

You May Not Need an Antibiotic If

- You do not have a history of frequent episodes of mastitis.

- You don't feel that sick.

- You have not gotten progressively sicker over the last few hours.

- Your fever is not rising.

- The breast pain and tenderness is not increasing.

- You can easily correct whatever factors may have set you up for engorgement in the first place.

You May Need Antibiotic Treatment If You

- Have a history of frequent mastitis.

- Have a fever that is rising.

- Are feeling progressively sicker as the hours go by.

- Have cracked nipples, allowing bacteria to get into your breast tissue more easily.

Which antibiotics are best? The type of bacteria involved in mastitis is usually *staphylococcus*, and the two safest and most effective classes of antibiotics against this organism are cloxacillins and cephalosporins. Other frequently prescribed antibiotics are Augmentin or erythromycin. All of these antibiotics are safe to take while breastfeeding. Even though you will feel better after a few days of taking antibiotics, be sure to complete the full course of antibiotics prescribed by your doctor (usually ten days); otherwise you run the risk of the mastitis returning. If you don't feel better after two or three days on antibiotics, call your doctor. He or she may wish to prescribe a different medication.

Section 32.5

Sore Nipples

"Sore Nipples," at www.askdrsears.com, undated, by Dr. William P. Sears ©
AskDrSears.com. Used with permission. Information about Dr. Sears can be
found at the end of this chapter or at www.askdrsears.com.

Sore nipples are not inevitable during the early days of breastfeeding. Painful feedings are a signal that something's not right and
you need to make a change.

What's Normal?

You can expect some tenderness in your nipples during the first
days of breastfeeding. As baby grasps the nipple and stretches the
breast tissue, you may feel a pulling sensation that is uncomfortable.
However, as baby begins to suck and your milk lets down, breastfeeding should become more comfortable. This initial soreness should
improve within two to four days after birth, if baby is positioned well
at the breast and is latched on properly.

If baby is having difficulty learning to latch on efficiently, you can
expect that your nipples will be sore. Pain that lasts throughout the
feeding or soreness that persists beyond one week postpartum indi-
cates that something needs to be changed about the way that baby is
latching on or sucking. It's important to do something about nipple
soreness before it gets worse and your nipples develop painful cracks.
If you are dreading the next feeding because your nipples hurt, get
some help from a lactation specialist.

Sore nipples in the first days and weeks postpartum are usually
the result of poor latch-on or baby's sucking technique. Sore nipples
that persist beyond the early weeks postpartum or that occur after
weeks or months of pain-free breastfeeding may have other causes,
such as a candida infection.

Preventing Sore Nipples

Careful attention to how your baby takes the breast will prevent,
or at least minimize, problems with sore nipples. Prevention is by far

the best cure! If you have problems with positioning and latch-on, get hands-on help from a lactation consultant before your nipples get terribly sore and your baby develops poor nursing habits.

What to Do about Sore Nipples: Fixing the Cause

The first and most important thing to do if you have sore nipples is to check how baby is being positioned at the breast and how baby is latching on. When baby is positioned and latched on correctly, the sucking pressure and the action of his tongue and gums is on the areola (the pigmented area around the nipple), rather than on the sensitive nipple itself.

If your nipples are very sore, baby is probably not getting enough breast tissue in his mouth. A horizontal red stripe across the tip of your nipple or a temporary indentation at the base of your nipple are signs that the nipple is not far enough back in the baby's mouth during sucking. The baby's tongue may be rubbing against the tip of the nipple (ouch!) or the baby's gums are chomping at the base of the nipple instead of on the areola over the milk sinuses. This kind of sucking is painful for mom, and inefficient for baby. Baby will not get enough milk if he sucks only the tip of your nipple. Here's how to work on the problem:

Review Latch-On Basics

- Is your baby well supported at the level of your nipple?
- Is she turned on her side and pulled close to the breast during feedings?
- Is she taking the breast with a wide open mouth?
- Are both her top and bottom lips turned out like a fish?
- Are your back, shoulders and arms well supported so that baby does not slip down onto the nipple as the feeding continues and you relax your hold on her?
- Are you supporting the breast with your fingers underneath, thumb on top, keeping the weight of the breast off baby's chin?

Encourage Baby to Take More Breast Tissue into Her Mouth

At least one inch (2.5 cm) of breast beyond the nipple should disappear into baby's mouth. Wait for baby to open her mouth very wide before pulling her in close to take the breast. Be sure that baby is latched on far enough back on the areola.

Try the "Breast Sandwich" to Help You Cram More Breast into Baby's Mouth

Support your breast with fingers underneath, thumb on top, well behind the areola. Press in with your thumb and fingers to flatten the breast while at the same time pushing back toward your chest. This makes the areola longer and narrower and easier for baby to take into his mouth.

Keep Baby's Mouth Open Wide

Use the index finger on the hand supporting the breast to push down on baby's chin as she latches on. You can continue putting gentle pressure on her chin throughout the feeding. Keeping her mouth open wide throughout the feeding should keep her from "tight mouthing" the breast. This will make breastfeeding more comfortable for you.

Make Sure Baby's Lips Are Turned Out

Sucking in the lower lip will cause soreness underneath the nipple. It's often hard for a mother to see if baby's lower lip is turned out when he is latched on, so ask someone else to peek under the breast and check this for you. You can gently pull baby's lip into a more comfortable position while he is latched on.

Check Baby's Tongue while Breastfeeding

If you gently pull down on baby's lower lip, you should be able to see the front of the tongue extended over the lower gum between the baby's lower lip and your areola. The tongue is cupped under the breast to help draw the milk from the reservoirs and channel it to the back of the mouth for swallowing. The tongue also protects the nipple from vigorous sucking. If you don't see baby's tongue under the breast during sucking, it may be pulled back and up in baby's mouth, where it will rub on the nipple causing soreness.

Correct the Position of the Tongue

Be sure that baby is taking the breast with a wide-open mouth and the tongue forward and down. To encourage baby to bring her tongue forward and down, use the index finger of the hand supporting the breast to press down gently on baby's chin during latch-on. Opening the jaw wider naturally causes the tongue to protrude further. Tucking baby's chin down before latch-on will also help to bring the tongue down when baby latches on. Breastfeeding in the clutch hold may also be helpful.

Consider the Possibility of Tongue-Tie

If it seems as if baby's tongue can't protrude over the lower gum, or if it seems to curl downward rather than cupping under the breast, or if it seems to push the breast out of baby's mouth, he may have a tongue thrust.

Always Break the Suction before Taking Baby off the Breast

"Popping" baby off the breast hurts, and leaves your nipples hurting for a surprisingly long time. Slip a clean finger into the corner of baby's mouth to release the suction before taking baby off the breast. Or, try pressing down gently on the breast near baby's mouth.

Avoid Artificial Nipples during the Time that Your Baby Is Learning to Breastfeed

Getting milk from bottles requires a different technique than breastfeeding. Using the bottle technique at the breast leads to latch-on and sucking problems. Babies who get both the bottle and breast in the early days are likely to have problems with nipple confusion. Avoid pacifiers as well as artificial nipples on feeding bottles.

In the early days of breastfeeding, you'll have to keep working at getting your baby latched on properly, even if it means taking the baby off the breast and starting over several times at the beginning of feedings. If you do this, you'll soon be rewarded with pain-free breastfeeding. If you are struggling with latch-on or your nipples have gone beyond the mildly sore stage to the painfully cracked or bleeding stage, get help. The sooner you get help, the easier it will be to fix the problem. Call a lactation consultant or a La Leche League Leader.

What to Do about Sore Nipples: Making Breastfeeding More Comfortable

Improving your baby's latch-on and sucking techniques will make breastfeeding more comfortable in the days to come. Realize this soreness won't last forever, and in a few days the pain should begin to lessen. To make breastfeeding less painful right now, try these suggestions:

Use Different Breastfeeding Positions

Try the cradle hold, the clutch hold, and the side-lying position. Varying positions from one feeding to the next changes the distribution of pressure on your areola and nipple during sucking.

Feed Baby on the Side That Is Least Sore First

Start the feeding on the less-tender breast. If you need to empty the sore breast, switch baby to that side after you have had a milk-ejection reflex. The pain from sore nipples is usually less intense after the milk is flowing.

Feed Baby before He Is Desperately Hungry

His sucking will be less vigorous and he can cooperate better with your latch-on lessons. Shorter, more frequent feedings are easier on your nipples than longer nursing sessions spaced farther apart.

Pad Your Nipple

As you're putting baby to the breast, use your thumb and index finger to slide the skin of the areola forward with gentle compression. This forms a wrinkle at the base of the nipple, which adds extra padding to protect the sore nipple.

Let Baby Suck on Your Index Finger Instead of a Pacifier

Long periods of comfort sucking at the end of feedings may be hard to endure. Use a well-scrubbed pinky finger if baby needs to suck for comfort and your nipples are wearing out. When baby sucks on an artificial pacifier, he learns sucking habits that will make it more difficult for him to learn to latch on and suck correctly at the breast. Sucking on an adult finger that extends well into baby's mouth is a better alternative in the early weeks of life.

Avoid Engorgement

It is more difficult for a baby to latch on to a breast that is swollen and engorged. Frequent feedings will help prevent this. While you may want to limit the amount of comfort sucking your baby does when your nipples are very sore, be sure that you breastfeed often enough and long enough for baby to get the milk out of your breasts. Engorgement can make problems with latch-on and sore nipples worse.

Numb Your Nipples

If your nipples are exquisitely tender, try numbing your nipples before breastfeeding by applying ice wrapped in a damp cloth.

Caring for Sore Nipples

You'll want to do everything you can to help your nipples feel better and heal quickly. Following are some time-tested tips for soothing tender nipple skin.

- After each feeding, manually express a few drops of milk and massage this natural skin-soother into the skin of your nipples. This stimulates circulation and promotes healing. Colostrum is an ideal nipple cream.

- Be sure the surface of your nipple is free of moisture when not in use. Pat your nipples dry with a soft cotton cloth after feedings. If patting hurts, let your nipples air dry. Leave your bra flaps down and your shirt open, if practical, until the nipple is no longer moist. Or, go without a bra, especially at night. You can sleep on a towel to absorb any leaking milk. Use fresh, dry breast pads without plastic liners after feedings to be sure no moisture stays in contact with your tender skin.

- Don't use quick drying methods, such as a hair dryer (even on a low setting), to dry your nipples. While some nipples tolerate this technique, it can cause more delicate nipples to crack because it dries the skin itself, not just the surface of the skin.

- Try exposing your nipples to a few minutes of sunshine during the day. Only two or three minutes, though, because sunburned nipples would be a disaster!

- To soothe and help heal sore nipples, use a modified lanolin ointment, such as Lansinoh. Massage a small amount into your nipples after nursing. Don't use oils or creams that are not safe for baby and would need to be washed off before breastfeeding. Medical-grade, modified lanolin works on the principle of moist wound healing, allowing the skin of the areola and nipple to retain its natural moisture. This prevents cracking and speeds up the process of healing.

- Avoid using soap on your nipples. The little bumps on the areola around your nipples are glands that secrete a natural cleansing and lubricating oil. Soaps remove these natural oils, causing dryness and cracking.

- Check your bra. Be sure your bra is not so tight that it compresses your nipples or so rough that it irritates them. Your nipples may feel better if you go without a bra and wear a soft T-shirt instead.

- If your nipples are too tender to touch, try wearing breast shells in your bra. These will hold the bra fabric away from your sore nipples and allow nothing but air to touch them. You can obtain breast shells through a lactation consultant, who will also help you determine the cause of your sore nipples and help resolve the problem.

When Nothing Else Is Working

If your nipples are still very sore after using the above measures, you may need to take more drastic action. If you haven't seen a lactation consultant yet, now is the time. You need expert help in fixing the cause of the soreness. A lactation consultant can show you how to teach your baby to suck better so that he will not traumatize your nipples. If your nipples really need a rest, try the following suggestions:

Try a Nipple Shield

This is a soft, flexible silicon artificial nipple that fits over your nipple and areola. The baby sucks on the shield to get milk out of the breast. Nipple shields can ease the pain during vigorous sucking and can also provide a temporary solution to some latch-on difficulties. Nipple shields, however, should be used with a great deal of caution. Studies show that babies get twenty to fifty percent less milk during sucking with a shield because they are unable to compress the milk sinuses beneath the areola very well. To lessen this problem, use only the new thin, soft, silicon shields. Be sure baby's lips are turned out and positioned high on the part of the shield that covers the areola, and not just on the nipple. Try to use the nipple shield only temporarily, since some babies develop problems with latch-on if these shields are overused. Also, long-term use of a nipple shield can lead to problems with your milk supply, since the breasts don't receive as much stimulation. To wean your baby from the shield, try using it only at the beginning of feedings. Once the baby is latched on and nursing, quickly slip the shield off and get baby attached directly to the breast. Eventually, baby will take the breast without the shield at the start of the feeding. You can obtain a nipple shield from a lactation consultant, who will also help you resolve the problems that have made the nipple shield necessary.

Rest the Breast with a Pump

Let baby suck on the nipple that is less sore while you pump the sore side for a day or so. But be careful. Pumping can irritate the nipples if you use too much suction, pump for too long, or if the nipple rubs against the flange of the pump. Offer the milk that you pump to your baby using a cup, a feeding syringe, or a spoon. Avoid giving supplements with artificial nipples. Feeding pumped milk with an artificial nipple will often make it more difficult to solve the latch-on problems that caused the sore nipples in the first place.

Consider Other Causes

If after trying all the above measures your nipples remain exquisitely tender, suspect a yeast infection, called candida. Sore nipples that appear after weeks or months of comfortable breastfeeding are almost always caused by yeast. Other causes of persistent sore nipples include eczema or Reynaud's syndrome.

About the Author

Dr. William Sears, M.D. is Associate Clinical Professor of Pediatrics at the University of California, Irvine, School of Medicine, and the co-author of numerous books on childbirth and parenting including *The Baby Book* (Little Brown & Co., 1992) and *The Breastfeeding Book* (Little Brown & Co., 2000). He is also a medical and parenting consultant for *BabyTalk* and *Parenting* magazines. Additional information about Dr. Sears can be found at www.askdrsears.com/aboutdrsears.asp.

Chapter 33

Tips to Increase Milk Supply

Many mothers wonder if their babies are getting enough to eat. Listed below are some of the signs that mean a breastfed baby is being well nourished:

- Your baby nurses eight to twelve times in twenty-four hours.

- Your baby acts relaxed and comfortable after eating.

- Your baby wets at least six cloth or five disposable diapers and has at least one bowel movement in twenty-four hours. The number of bowel movements may change after the first few weeks.

- You can hear your baby swallow milk while nursing.

- Your breasts seem softer after nursing.

- Your baby gains four to seven ounces a week after the first week. There is no need to weigh your baby at home, your baby's doctor will do this for you.

It is not a good idea to offer a bottle of water or formula after nursing to see if your baby is still hungry. Most babies will suck on a bottle after nursing. This just means they need to suck. It does not mean

"Breast-feeding: Tips to Increase Your Milk Supply," Patient Information Sheet 162. University Hospitals Health System, University Hospitals of Cleveland. ©1992, revised 1998. Used with permission.

they are still hungry. Babies cry or fuss for many reasons, such as being tired, bored, wet, hot, or cold.

Beginning birth control pills too soon can decrease your milk supply. It is best to wait at least six weeks before beginning birth control pills. Then use only the mini-pill called Progestin. If you still notice a decrease in your milk supply, discuss other birth control options with your doctor.

Smoking can also contribute to a decreased milk supply. If you can't stop smoking:

- Try to cut down.

- Smoke after nursing.

- Don't smoke in the same room with your baby.

If your baby shows signs of needing more nourishment, you can do the following to increase your milk supply:

- Nurse your baby every two hours during the day and every three to four hours at night (at least eight to twelve times in twenty-four hours).

- Feed your baby at least fifteen minutes at each breast. Allow him to decide if he needs to nurse longer. Do not limit nursing time.

- Nurse your baby at both breasts at each feeding. If baby falls asleep, wake him to change breasts.

- Do not supplement your baby's feedings with formula, water, or baby food. Usually, no other foods are necessary for six months if you are exclusively breastfeeding.

- Drink plenty of fluids so that your urine is very pale in color.

- Eat high-protein foods.

- Take your iron supplement if your health care provider says you are anemic.

- Discuss the need for vitamin and lecithin supplements with your doctor or nurse-midwife.

- Take a nap whenever your baby sleeps.

- Do not use nipple shields or pacifiers.

Some mothers have reported success with increasing milk production by:

- Drinking two nonalcoholic beers per day.

- Taking two brewer's yeast tablets per day.

- Taking the herb fenugreek—two capsules, three times per day. (Talk to your doctor first. Fenugreek can lower blood glucose levels in diabetic mothers, can sometimes cause diarrhea in mothers, and can aggravate asthma symptoms in asthmatic mothers.) As a rule, milk production increases within seventy-two hours after starting fenugreek.

Chapter 34

Breast Compression: Assisting the Flow of Milk

The purpose of breast compression is to continue the flow of milk to the baby once the baby no longer drinks (open-pause-close type of suck) on his own. Breast compression simulates a letdown reflex and often stimulates a natural letdown reflex to occur. The technique may be useful for:

- Poor weight gain in the baby
- Colic in the breastfed baby
- Frequent feedings and/or long feedings
- Sore nipples in the mother
- Recurrent blocked ducts and/or mastitis
- Encouraging the baby who falls asleep quickly to continue drinking

Breast compression is not necessary if everything is going well. When all is going well, the mother should allow the baby to finish feeding on the first side and, if the baby wants more, should offer the other side. How do you know the baby is finished? When he no longer drinks at the breast (open-pause-close type of suck).

From Handout #15 by Jack Newman, M.D., F.R.C.P. Revised January 1998. ©1998 by Promotion of Mother's Milk (ProMoM, Inc.), www.ProMoM.com. Reprinted with permission.

A baby who is latched on well gets milk more easily than one who is not. A baby who is poorly latched on can get milk only when the flow of milk is rapid. Thus, many mothers and babies do well with breastfeeding in spite of a poor latch because most mothers produce an abundance of milk.

In the first three to six weeks of life, babies fall asleep at the breast when the flow of milk is slow, not necessarily when they have had enough to eat. After this age, they may start to pull away at the breast when the flow of milk slows down.

Unfortunately many babies are latching on poorly. If the mother's supply is abundant the baby often does well as far as weight gain is concerned, but the mother may pay a price—sore nipples, a colicky baby, or a baby who is constantly on the breast but feeding only a small part of the time.

Breast compression continues the flow of milk once the baby starts falling asleep at the breast and results in the baby not only getting more milk, but getting more milk that is high in fat.

Breast Compression: How to Do It

1. Hold the baby with one arm.

2. Hold the breast with the other hand, thumb on one side of the breast, your other fingers on the other, fairly far back from the nipple.

3. Watch for the baby's drinking, though there is no need to be obsessive about catching every suck. The baby gets substantial amounts of milk when he is drinking with an open-pause-close type of suck. Open-pause-close is one suck, the pause is not a pause between sucks.

4. When the baby is nibbling or no longer drinking with the open-pause-close type of suck, compress the breast, but not so hard that it hurts. Try not to change the shape of the areola (the part of the breast near the baby's mouth). With the compression, the baby should start drinking again with the open-pause-close type of suck.

5. Keep the pressure up until the baby no longer drinks even with the compression, then release the pressure. Often the baby will stop sucking altogether when the pressure is released, but will start again shortly as milk starts to flow

again. If the baby does not stop sucking with the release of pressure, wait a short time before compressing again.

6.   The reason to release the pressure is to allow your hand to rest, and to allow milk to start flowing to the baby again. The baby, if he stops sucking when you release the pressure, will start again when he starts to taste milk.

7.   When the baby starts sucking again, he may drink (open-pause-close). If not, compress again as above.

8.   Continue on the first side until the baby does not drink even with the compression. You should allow the baby to stay on the side for a short time longer, as you may occasionally get another letdown reflex and the baby will start drinking again on his own. If the baby no longer drinks, however, allow him to come off or take him off the breast.

9.   If the baby wants more, offer the other side and repeat the process.

10.   You may wish, unless you have sore nipples, to switch sides back and forth in this way several times.

11.   Work on improving the baby's latch.

The above works best, but if you find a way which works better at keeping the baby sucking with an open-pause-close type of suck, use whatever works best for you and your baby. As long as it does not hurt your breast to compress, and as long as the baby is drinking (open-pause-close type of suck), breast compression is working.

You will not always need to do this. As breastfeeding improves, you will able to let things happen naturally.

Chapter 35

The Use of Reglan® to Increase Milk Supply

Occasionally mothers may have difficulty establishing or maintaining breastmilk production. This may occur when a mother is:

- Ill.

- Pumping breastmilk for an extended period to feed a premature or ill newborn.

- Weaning temporarily, then restarting breastfeeding.

- Nursing an adopted infant.

- Nursing after breast surgery.

Reglan® (Metoclopramide) is a drug used in infants, children, and adults to improve upper gastrointestinal function. In infants, it is often used to treat gastroesophageal reflux (vomiting). In children and adults, it is used to treat heartburn, and to treat the nausea and vomiting caused by other drugs.

Reglan® (Metoclopramide) has, as a side effect, the ability to increase prolactin, the milk-making hormone in the brain. Prolactin, along with frequent and regular breast pumping, increases breastmilk production.

"The Use of Reglan® (Metoclopramide) to Increase Milk Supply" © 1995 San Diego County Breastfeeding Coalition. Reprinted with permission of San Diego County Breastfeeding Coalition, http://www.breastfeeding.org. Reviewed and revised by David A. Cooke, M.D. on October 14, 2001.

183

Reglan® (Metoclopramide) is usually taken as a 10 mg tablet orally, three or four times a day for a week, then tapered off over the next week. Cost for thirty tablets is approximately $33 for the brand name Reglan®, and $12–15 for the generic brand, which is just as effective. Milk supply usually increases within two to four days of starting the medication and pumping six to eight times per twenty-four hours. It is essential that the milk be emptied frequently from the breasts, even at night.

Although Reglan® (Metoclopramide) can be safely given to infants, a small amount of mother's dose will get into the milk. Studies have shown no infant side effects, but watch for sleepiness and poor feeding in your infant.

Side effects may occur in a small number of mothers. Restlessness, drowsiness, fatigue, and diarrhea may occur, but usually do not require stopping the medication. Driving while taking the medication may not be wise if you are feeling fatigued. Rare side effects are sleeplessness, headache, confusion, dizziness, mental depression, feelings of anxiety, and agitation. If you have any of these, discontinue the drug. A very rare side effect (less than one per five hundred people taking the drug) is an "acute dystonic reaction" where you have difficulty controlling your muscle movements, including your eye movements. Discontinue the drug and call your physician. Benedryl® (diphenhydramine) will stop this reaction.

Reglan® (Metoclopramide) should NOT be used if you:

- Have epilepsy or are on anti-seizure medications.

- Have a history of mental depression or are on antidepressant drugs.

- Have a tumor called a Pheochromocytoma or uncontrolled high blood pressure.

- Have intestinal bleeding or obstruction.

- Have a known allergy or prior reaction to Reglan® (Metoclopramide).

Reglan® (metoclopramide) can interact with a number of medications. If you are taking other medications (prescription, nonprescription, or herbal), you should bring all of them to your physician's attention before starting a prescription for Reglan® (Metoclopramide).

While Reglan® (metoclopramide) is generally the preferred medication when one is considered necessary to augment milk supply, some other agents have also been used successfully. Thorazine® (chlorpromazine) may also work, but is rarely used due to serious side effects. Traditionally, a number of herbal agents have also been used, including preparations of Fenugreek seed, fennel seed, and milk thistle. Unfortunately, very little data is available on how well they work compared to other agents. Additionally, there is almost no information on their safety for mother or infant; "natural" remedies are not necessarily any safer than prescription drugs.

For further information, or if you have any concerns, consult your, or your baby's physician.

References

1. Budd SS, Erdman SH, Long DM et al: Improved lactation with metoclopramide: A case report. *Clin Pediatr* 1993;32:53.

2. Ehrenkrantz RA, Ackerman BA: Metoclopramide effect on faltering milk production by mothers of premature infants. *Pediatrics* 1986;78:614.

3. Gupta AP, Gupta PK: Metoclopramide as a lactogogue. *Clin Pediatr* 1985;24(5):269–272.

4. Lawrence RA: *Breastfeeding: A Guide for the Medical Profession*, ed4, St Louis, Mosby, 1994.

5. *Physicians' Desk Reference*, ed 49, Montvale, NJ, Medical Economics, 1995.

Chapter 36

Colic in the Breastfed Baby

Colic is one of the mysteries of nature. Nobody knows what it really is, but everyone has an opinion. In the typical situation, the baby starts to have crying periods about two to three weeks after birth. These occur mainly in the evening, and finally stop when the baby is about three months of age (occasionally older). When the baby cries, he is often inconsolable; however, if he is walked, rocked, or taken for a drive he may settle temporarily. For a baby to be called colicky, it is necessary that he be gaining weight well and be otherwise healthy.

The notion of colic has been extended to include almost any fussiness or crying in the baby, and this may be valid since we do not really know what colic is. There is no treatment for colic, though many medications and behavior strategies have been tried without any proven benefit. It is admitted that everyone knows someone whose baby was cured of colic by a particular treatment. It is also admitted that almost every treatment seems to work—for a short time, anyhow.

There are three known situations in the breastfed baby which may result in fussiness or colic. Once again, it is assumed that the baby is gaining adequately and that the baby is healthy.

Feeding Both Breasts at Each Feeding

Human milk changes during a feeding. One of the ways in which it changes is that the amount of fat increases as the baby nurses longer

Handout 2, "Colic in the Breastfed Baby" by Jack Newman, M.D., F.R.C.P.C. Revised 1998, reprinted with permission.

187

at the breast. If the mother automatically switches the baby from one breast to the other during the feed, before the baby has finished the first side, the baby may get a relatively low amount of fat during the feeding. This may result in the baby getting fewer calories, and thus feeding more frequently. If the baby takes in a lot of milk (to make up for the reduced concentration of calories), he may spit up. Because of the relatively low fat content of the milk, the stomach empties quickly, and a large load of milk sugar (lactose) arrives in the intestine all at once. The protein which digests the sugar (lactase) may not be able to handle so much milk sugar at one time and the baby will have the symptoms of lactose intolerance—crying; gas; and explosive, watery, greenish bowel movements. This may occur even during the feeding. These babies are not lactose intolerant. They have problems with lactose because of the sort of information women get about breastfeeding. This is not a reason to switch to lactose-free formula.

What Can Be Done?

- Do not time feedings. Mothers all over the world have breastfed babies successfully without being able to tell time. Breastfeeding problems are greatest in societies where everyone has a watch and least where no one has a watch.

- The mother should feed the baby on one breast, as long as the baby breastfeeds (until the baby comes off himself or is asleep at the breast). If the baby feeds for only a short time only, the mother can compress the to keep the baby nursing. Please note that a baby may be on the breast for two hours, but may actually feed for only a few minutes. In that case the milk taken by the baby may still be relatively low in fat. This is the rationale for compressing the breast. If, after finishing on the first side, the baby still wants to feed, offer the other side.

- The next feeding, the mother should start the baby on the other breast in the same way. The mother's body will adjust quickly to the new method, and she will not become engorged or lopsided.

- Just as there should be no rule for feeding both breasts at each feeding, there should be no rule for one breast per feeding. Let the baby finish on one breast (compress milk into his mouth if necessary to keep him swallowing longer) but if he wants more, then offer the other side.

- In some cases, it may be helpful to feed the baby two or more feedings on one side before switching over to the other side for two or more feedings.

- This problem is made worse if the baby is not well latched on to the breast. A proper latch is the key to easy breastfeeding.

Overactive Let-Down Reflex

A baby who gets too much milk too quickly may become very fussy and very irritable at the breast, and may be considered colicky. Typically, the baby is gaining very well. Typically, also, the baby starts nursing, and after a few seconds or minutes, starts to cough, choke, or struggle at the breast. He may come off, and often, the mother's milk will spray. After this, the baby frequently returns to the breast, but may be fussy and repeat the performance. He may be unhappy with the rapid flow, and impatient when the flow slows. This can be a very trying time for everyone. On rare occasions, a baby may even start refusing to take the breast after several weeks, typically around three months of age.

What Can Done?

- If you have not already done so, try feeding the baby one breast per feed. In some situations, feeding even two or three feedings on one breast before changing to the other breast may be helpful. If you experience engorgement on the unused breast, express just enough to feel comfortable.

- Feed the baby before he is ravenous. Do not hold off the feeding by giving water (a breastfeeding baby does not need water even in very hot weather) or a pacifier. A ravenous baby will "attack" the breast and cause a very active letdown reflex. Feed the baby as soon as he shows any sign of hunger. If he is still half asleep, all the better.

- Feed the baby in a calm, relaxed, atmosphere, if possible. Loud music, bright lights, and lots of action are not conducive to a successful feeding.

- Lying down to nurse sometimes works very well. If lying sideways to feed does not help, try lying flat on your back with the baby lying on top of you to nurse. Gravity helps decrease the flow rate.

189

- If you have time, express some milk (an ounce or so) before you feed the baby.

- The baby may dislike the rapid flow, but also become fussy when the flow slows too much. If you think the baby is fussy because the flow is too slow, it will help to compress the breast to keep up the flow.

- This problem is made worse if the baby is not well latched on to the breast. A good latch is the key to easy breastfeeding.

- On occasion giving the baby two to four drops of commercial lactase (the enzyme that metabolizes lactose) before each feeding relieves the symptoms. It is available without prescription, but it is fairly expensive and works only occasionally.

- A nipple shield may help, but use this only if nothing else has helped and only if you have gotten good help without any relief.

- As a last resort, rather than switching to formula, give the baby your expressed milk by bottle.

Foreign Proteins in the Mother's Milk

It has been shown that some proteins present in the mother's diet may be excreted into her milk and may affect the baby. It would seem that the most common of these is cow's milk protein. Other proteins have also been shown to be excreted into some mothers' milk. The fact that these proteins and other substances appear in the mother's milk is not necessarily a bad thing. Indeed, it should be considered a good thing. Ask about this if you have any questions.

Thus, in the treatment of the colicky breastfed baby, one step would be for the mother to stop eating dairy products. These includes milk, cheese, yogurt, ice cream, and anything else which may contain milk. When the milk protein has been changed (denatured), as when cooked, there should be no problem. Ask if you have any questions.

Please note: Intolerance to milk protein has nothing to do with lactose intolerance. A mother who is herself lactose intolerant should also still breastfeed her baby.

What Can Be Done?

- The mother should eliminate all milk products for seven to ten days.

- If there has been no change, the mother can reintroduce milk products.

- If there has been a change for the better, the mother should then slowly reintroduce milk products into her diet, if these are normally part of her diet. There is no need to drink milk in order to make milk. Some babies tolerate absolutely no milk products in the mother's diet. Most tolerate some. The mother will learn what amount of dairy products she can take without the baby reacting. Ask if you have any questions. One week off milk products will not cause any problems. Actually, evidence suggests that breastfeeding may protect the woman against the development of osteoporosis even if she does not take extra calcium, and the baby will get all he needs.

- The mother should be careful about eliminating too many things from her diet. Everyone will know someone whose baby got better when the mother stopped broccoli, beef, bananas, bread, etc. The mother may find that she is eating white rice only. Our diets are too complex to be sure exactly what, if anything, is affecting the baby.

Be patient, the problem usually gets better no matter what. Formula is not the answer; however, because of the more regular flow some babies do improve on it. But formula is not breastmilk. In fact, the baby would also improve on breastmilk from the bottle because of the regularity of the flow. Even if nothing works, time usually helps. The days and nights may seem eternal, but the weeks will fly by.

Chapter 37

Allergies and Breastfeeding

Allergies today are more common than ever before—one in five children now shows some degree of allergy by age twenty. The incidence of allergies has increased tenfold over the past twenty years. This is partly due to increased exposure to known allergens (allergy-causing substances). It is also because physicians and allergy sufferers are more likely to recognize that certain symptoms or illnesses are caused by allergies (Lawrence 1994). Changes in the human diet from the days of hunter-gatherers eating seasonal foods to the year round availability of most foods has, surprisingly, reduced the number of foods in a typical diet from around 200 to just about 20. Narrowing food choices in this manner increases exposure to these foods and predisposes people to food allergies.

The earlier and more often a food is ingested, the greater likelihood it has of becoming an allergen. Babies tend to be most allergic to the foods they have been offered first. While a baby is exclusively breastfed, he is only exposed to the foods his mother eats and secretes in her milk, so his exposure to potential allergens is minimized.

One long-term study of children who were breastfed showed that breastfeeding reduces food allergies at least through adolescence (Grasky 1982). Protection from allergies is one of the most important benefits of breastfeeding. The incidence of cow's milk allergies is up

Excerpted from "Allergies and the Breastfeeding Family" by Karen Zeretzke. *New Beginnings* July-August 1998. Used with permission of La Leche League International (http://www.lalecheleague.org).

Table 37.1. Possible Symptoms of Allergy

Gastrointestinal System

Vomiting, spitting up

Diarrhea

Blood in stools

Colic

Occult bleeding

Cramping

Constipation

Gas

Malabsorption (and resulting poor weight gain)

Colitis

Protein and iron-losing enteropathy

Neonatal thrombocytopenia (low levels of platelets in the blood)

Respiratory System

Runny nose

Sneezing

Coughing

Rattling

Asthma

Red, itchy nose (allergic salute)

Pulmonary disorders

Bronchitis

Congestion, prolonged cold-like symptoms

Recurrent nosebleed

Mouth breathing

Stridor (noisy breathing)

Eyes

Swollen eyelids

Red eyes

Dark circles under eyes

Constant tearing of eyes

Gelatin-like fluid in eyes

Skin

Eczema

Dermatitis

Urticaria (hives)

Rash

Sore bottom

Redness around rectum

Itching

Flushed cheeks

Excessive pallor

Central Nervous System

Irritability

Fussiness

Sleeplessness

Light sleeper

Restlessness

Prolonged drowsiness

Other Symptoms

Ear infections

Hiccoughs

Poor weight gain

Excessive drooling

Excessive sweating

Aching in legs and other muscles

Short attention span

Poor school performance

Hard to live with

Depression

Spots on tongue

Failure-to-thrive

Swelling of lips, tongue, throat

Life-threatening drop in blood pressure

to seven times greater in babies who are fed artificial baby milk instead of human milk (Lawrence 1994).

Breastfeeding protects against allergies in two ways. The first and most obvious reason breastfed babies have fewer allergies is that they are exposed to fewer allergens in the first months of life. They aren't given formula based cow's milk or soy products. Less exposure to these foods means less chance of allergy later on. The other reason breastfed babies have fewer allergies has to do with the development of the immune system. At birth, a baby's immune system is immature. Babies depend heavily on antibodies obtained from their mothers while in the womb. Their digestive systems are not really ready for substances other than their mothers' milk. At about six weeks of age, Pyer's Patches in the intestines begin to produce immunoglobulins or antibodies. At six months of age, a baby has a functional, if immature, immune system that is capable of producing secretory immunoglobulin A (sIgA), the antibody found in all body secretions that is the first line of defense against foreign substances.

In the meantime, a baby depends on mother's milk for protection. Fed from his mother's breast, a baby first receives colostrum, the first milk, which is especially rich in antibodies, including sIgA. The sIgA "paints" a protective coating on the inside of a baby's intestines to prevent penetration by potential allergens. Mature milk continues to provide this "protection-from-the-inside" to help the baby remain healthy and allergy free. Human milk and colostrum also provide antibodies specifically designed to fight germs to which either the mother or baby has been exposed.

The tendency to be allergic is often inherited from a child's mother or father. Babies with a family history of allergy seem to have different immune responses than those without allergies.

How Allergies Occur

Allergies happen when a person's body perceives a normally harmless substance (such as pollen, mold, dust, or a particular food) as an invader. In its own defense, the body produces large amounts of the antibody immunoglobulin E (IgE). When the antibodies come in contact with the substance the body perceives as dangerous, they attach themselves to tissue and blood cells. These cells then release powerful inflammatory chemicals, called mediators: histamines, prostaglandins, and leukotrienes. These in turn affect mucous glands, capillaries, and smooth muscles, causing the sufferer to experience allergic symptoms.

195

Symptoms are usually found in more than one body system and can be downright contradictory. Reactions to food most commonly cause symptoms in the gastrointestinal system, including spitting up, diarrhea (in a breastfed infant, this means stools are looser, more watery, and greater in number and volume than usual), cramping, constipation, gas, malabsorption of nutrients (which could result in poor weight gain), and colitis. The respiratory system, skin, eyes, and central nervous system may also be involved in allergic reactions to food. Table 37.1 gives an idea of what form allergic symptoms can take. Generally more than one body system is involved in an allergic reaction. Gastrointestinal symptoms are most common.

Parents often use behavior to help identify allergies in their child. How a child feels will be revealed in behavior. A child who doesn't feel well can't behave well. A baby whose body chemistry is muddled by allergies will be confused and miserable.

Common Allergy-Causing Foods

Cow's Milk Tops the List

Lists of the foods most likely to trigger allergic responses differ from source to source and culture to culture, but cow's milk and dairy products top them all. There are more than 20 substances in cow's milk that have been shown to be human allergens (Stigler 1985). Colic and vomiting are often caused by cow's milk allergy. Eczema—dry, rough, red skin patches which can progress to open, weeping sores—is another common symptom among children allergic to cow's milk. Cow's milk has been found to cause sleeplessness in infants and toddlers. Dairy allergy has also been suggested as a cause of bed wetting in an older child.

When fed cow's milk-based formulas, some babies react simply because of the large amounts of cow's milk they receive. Feeding a baby artificial baby milk is equivalent to an adult drinking seven quarts (almost eight liters) of milk a day! Allergies such as these are not accompanied by changes in the immune system—there is no rise in IgE levels—and they often subside spontaneously. Parents who are bottle feeding keep switching brands of formula until they find one that works or until the baby outgrows the symptoms.

Early and occasional exposure to cow's milk proteins can sensitize a baby so that even tiny amounts of cow's milk may trigger a response: IgE levels rise and a severe reaction may occur. Thus, sensitive babies may react to cow's milk in their mothers' diet. Small amounts of cow's milk protein may appear in a mother's milk and provoke a response in her baby, even if the mother herself is not allergic to cow's milk. If there is a family history of milk allergies, a mother may prefer to avoid dairy products in her diet as well as not offering them directly to her baby. Severe reactions could otherwise occur.

Other Culprits

Other common foods which cause allergic reactions are eggs, wheat, corn, pork, fish and shellfish, peanuts, tomatoes, onions, cabbage, berries, nuts, spices, citrus fruits and juices, and chocolate.

Some allergy sufferers have been helped by avoiding foods which have been exposed to chemicals while being grown or raised. Other things to consider avoiding include additives, flavorings, preservatives, and colorings. In many places, cows, pigs, and chickens are fed antibiotics to produce healthy animals; these may cause or trigger allergies in very susceptible individuals. Coatings on vitamins or other medications can cause an allergic response, as can fluoride, iron, and some herbal preparations. Be sure no siblings or other family members are giving the baby a taste of anything—this is one time when sharing is not appropriate. Eating foods that are chilled or cold sets off reactions for some.

Sometimes mothers feel that because a food could be a potential allergen, it is best to avoid it entirely. If there is no history of allergy to these foods in the mother's or father's family, this may be an unnecessary precaution. Eating foods a mother enjoys will help her to find breastfeeding more satisfying. Mothers do not have to give up foods they love while breastfeeding. Only if a baby shows allergic symptoms should a mother consider avoiding certain foods.

Treating Allergies

A Detective Game

There is no cure for allergies. The easiest and least expensive treatment for many who suffer from allergies to foods is simply to avoid those foods.

Discovering exactly which foods a baby reacts to can be a difficult process, but is well worth the effort. For a breastfed baby, this might involve keeping a record of foods eaten by the mother along with notes on the baby's symptoms and behavior. Over time, it is usually possible to see connections between certain foods and a baby's distress. If highly allergic, babies can react to foods their mothers have eaten within minutes, although symptoms generally show up between four and twenty-four hours after exposure. The mother then may develop an eating plan for herself which eliminates suspected foods. If this produces a happier baby, the mother can then challenge her findings by eating some of the suspected food. A repeated reaction from the baby confirms his sensitivity to this food, and his mother may well choose to limit or avoid it for some time.

Most babies will show distinct improvement after an allergenic food has been removed from the mother's diet for five to seven days, but it may take two weeks or more to totally eliminate all traces of the offending substance from both the mother and her baby. Elimination diets can be time consuming; however, many mothers find they are worth the effort.

Rotation Diets

Many mothers have found that following a rotation diet permits them to eat even foods to which the baby has reacted (Stigler 1985). A rotation diet allows troublesome foods to be eaten in a rotating schedule so that there is a three to seven day gap in between days the food is eaten. This allows a food to be completely eliminated from the mother's body before she ingests it again, which can prevent allergic symptoms from developing in her baby. The stronger the baby's reaction to the food, the longer the mother should go before exposing the baby to it again. Trial and error will permit the mother to make the best choice for her circumstances.

Foods that cause problems in babies often bother their mothers as well, but so much more subtly that the mothers are unaware until eliminating a food makes both mother and baby feel better, Ironically, foods that the mother craves and eats on a daily basis often fall into this category.

When a child begins eating solids, some mothers experience dermatitis or eczema on their nipples which may be caused by a food her baby or toddler is eating or medications he may be taking. Residuals of that substance in his mouth may cause reactions on the mother's skin.

Other Options

Other treatment options for allergies include medication, immunotherapy, and allergy tests. These can be particularly helpful when the allergen is one not easily avoided, such as pollen, dust, and environmental allergens.

Changing the child's environment by stripping his room to the bare walls and floor will often help an allergic child; the results have been likened to a military barracks look. No curtains, bedspreads, fluffy quilts, dust ruffles, carpeting, rugs, shutters, blinds, upholstered furniture, stuffed animals (except those which are hypoallergenic on both the outside and the inside), or furred or feathered pets. Shades may be used on the windows; pillows should be synthetic; blankets should be cotton or synthetic and should be washed weekly; mattress and box springs should be encased in plastic and furniture should be plain wood or plastic. The closet should hold only the clothes for the current season—no stored items. The space under the bed should be kept empty. Heating/air conditioning vents can be covered in muslin "shower caps" for easy removal and washing. Walls, woodwork, and furniture should be scrubbed at least every three months. If a vaporizer is used, it must be kept scrupulously clean. Some families have found air cleaning machines worth the investment.

Changing to unscented soaps and laundry powders and avoiding other products with additives, such as hair sprays, deodorants, disposable diapers and wipes, and other personal hygiene products has helped some families. Avoiding fumes and odors where possible, such as those from gas (both fuel for automobiles and cooking and heating fuel), paint, pesticides, chemicals, exhausts, insulation materials, new carpeting, and hay and other dried harvest products may also help.

Prevention for Subsequent Children

Once a family has experienced an allergic child, parents want to avoid allergy problems for subsequent children. Studies have shown that if a mother avoids all foods to which any members of her family show sensitivity during her entire pregnancy and period of lactation, later children are far less likely to have allergic symptoms (Chandra 1989). Avoiding eating any food in large amounts during pregnancy will lessen the likelihood of infant allergies to that food.

A pregnant woman who avoids cow's milk products must be sure to get adequate calcium from other sources, either through her diet or a calcium supplement. Ruth Lawrence recommends reagent quality powdered calcium carbonate (Lawrence 1994). Dietary sources of calcium include calcium-enriched tofu, collards, spinach, broccoli, turnip greens, kale, liver, almonds and Brazil nuts, as well as canned sardines and salmon.

Mothers who avoid potential allergens during pregnancy seem to have a lower incidence of pre-eclampsia, swelling, and yeast infections.

They also have less trouble with runny noses during pregnancy (Stigler 1985). These benefits to mothers may help compensate for giving up foods they may enjoy.

Pregnant mothers may also wish to stay inside on days when the pollen count is high. Research shows there is a seasonal clustering of higher miscarriages, late-pregnancy bleeding, extreme swelling, and ectopic pregnancies during hay fever season; and 10 days after an elevated ragweed count, hospitals admit more women with toxemia of pregnancy (Stigler 1985).

Although taking steps to reduce exposure to allergens may be tedious and difficult, the results are rewarding. It's extraordinary to see a child change from a whiny, irritable, aggressive, rash-prone, doesn't-know-what-he-wants, non-sleeper to a pleasant, clear-skinned, easy-going child who sleeps well. Once parents are confronted with this dramatic change, they are willing to do what it takes to help their child.

Resources

Books

1. Crook W: *Tracking Down Hidden Food Allergies*. Jackson, Tennessee, Professional Books, 1978.

2. Crook W: *You and Allergy*. Jackson, Tennessee, Professional Books, 1984.

3. La Leche League International: *The Womanly Art of Breastfeeding*. Schaumburg, Illinois, LLLI, 1997.

4. Lawrence R: *Breastfeeding: A Guide for the Medical Profession, ed 4*. St. Louis, Mosby, 1994.

5. Mohrbacher N, Stock J: *The Breastfeeding Answer Book*. Schaumburg, Illinois, LLLI, 1997.

6. Rapp D: *Is This Your Child?* New York, William Morrow and Company, Inc., 1991.

7. Rapp D: *Sneezing, Wheezing and Scratching*. Los Altos, California, The ECR Collection, 1974.

8. Riordan J, Auerbach K: *Breastfeeding and Human Lactation*. Boston, Massachusetts, Jones and Bartlett, 1993.

Periodical Articles

1. Blair H: Natural history of childhood asthma: A 20-year follow-up. *Arch Dis Child* 1977;52:613–619.

2. Chandra R, Puri S, Hamed A: Influence of maternal diet during lactation and use of formula feeds on development of atopic eczema in high risk infants. *Br Med J* 1989;299:228–30.

3. Gerrard J: Food allergy: Two common types as seen in breast and formula fed babies. *Ann Allergy* 1983;50:375–79.

4. Gruskay F: Comparison of breast, cow and soy feedings in the prevention of onset of allergic disease: A 15-year prospective study. *Clin Pediatr* 1982;21(8):486–91.

5. Host A, Husby S, Osterballe O: A prospective study of cow's milk allergy in exclusively breastfed infants. *Acta Paediatr Scand* 1988;77:663–70.

6. Jandl A:. Allergies. *New Beginnings* Mar-Apr1996;40–41.

7. Kahn A, Mozin M., Casimir C, et al: Insomnia and cow's milk allergy in infants. *Pediatrics*, 1985;76:880–85.

8. Lesniewski L: Coping with allergies. *New Beginnings* Sept-Oct 1988;140–142.

9. Merrett T, et al: Infant feeding and allergy: Twelve-month prospective study of 500 babies born into allergic families. *Ann Allergy* 1988;61:13.

10. Mohrbacher N: Reducing the risk of allergies. *New Beginnings* Sept-Oct 1988;143–44.

11. Saarinen L, Kajosaari M: Breastfeeding as prophylaxis against atopic disease: Prospective follow-up study until 17 years old. *Lancet* 1995;346:1065–69.

12. Sehee C: Late solids and allergies. *New Beginnings* Sept-Oct 1988;142–43.

13. Shircliff S: Bottoms up. *New Beginnings* Mar-Apr 1995;43–44.

14. Stigler U: Preventive dietary management: Prenatal, neonatal and in infancy. *Clin Ecol* 1985;3:1:50–54.

15. Sutin K: Eliminating foods worked wonders. *New Beginnings* Sept-Oct 1988;145.

Chapter 38

Thrush

What Is Thrush?

In the proper balance, yeast can be beneficial to our bodies. But when it becomes too abundant, problems such as thrush can develop, making breastfeeding painful. *Candida albicans*, the organism that causes thrush, is a fungus that thrives on milk on the nipples, in the milk ducts, and in the baby's mouth.

In the baby, possible symptoms of thrush include:

- diaper rash

- white patches on the inside of the mouth, cheeks, or tongue

- refusing the breast or a reluctance to nurse (because baby's mouth is sore).

The baby may also be without symptoms. In other words, a mother may have thrush on her nipples even if her baby has no sign of it.

In the mother, possible symptoms of thrush include:

- prolonged or sudden onset of sore nipples during or after the newborn period;

Excerpted from "Thrush" by Nancy Morhrbacher, *New Beginnings*, May-June 1993. Reprinted with permission of La Leche League International (LLLI), www.lalecheleague.org. Reviewed and revised by David A. Cooke, M.D. October 14, 2001.

- nipples that are pink, flaky, crusty, and itchy;

- nipples that are red and burning;

- cracked nipples; or

- a vaginal yeast (monilial) infection.

An intense stabbing or burning pain in one or both breasts during or shortly after feedings may mean that a secondary yeast infection has developed within the milk ducts. This seems to be more common if mother or baby has been on antibiotics (because antibiotics kill the beneficial bacteria in the body that keep yeast under control) or if the mother has had cracked nipples (the fungus can enter the breast through the cracks).

Thrush is more likely to develop if either mother or baby has been treated with antibiotics, the mother's diet is high in sugars, the mother has diabetes, or the mother's resistance is low due to fatigue or other health problems.

Although thrush is usually not serious, it can definitely be a nuisance. In a few reported cases, mothers have chosen to wean their babies because of the severity and persistence of thrush. Before reaching that point, however, a number of steps can be taken to solve the problem. Fortunately, the treatment for thrush need not interfere with nursing.

Treating Thrush

The first step in treating thrush is to contact a health-care provider. Mother and baby need to be treated simultaneously for at least two weeks, and breastfeeding need not be affected. In *Breastfeeding: A Guide for the Medical Profession*, Ruth Lawrence, M.D., recommends doctors prescribe liquid nystatin for the baby's mouth and a nystatin cream for the mother to apply to her nipples and areolae (the dark areas around the nipples). Nystatin pills or liquid for the mother may be necessary if deep breast pain develops or if the thrush recurs after a full course of treatment. Some strains of thrush have become resistant to nystatin, so if the nystatin does not bring relief, other drugs may be necessary. Topical clotrimazole cream is frequently recommended for use on the mother's nipples, but is not used for treating the infant. Over-the-counter preparations and other prescription drugs are available and may be used on the recommendation of a health-care professional.

In mild cases of thrush, once treatment has begun relief may be felt in twenty-four to forty-eight hours. In severe cases, the symptoms may take three to five days to disappear. It is important that the medication be continued for the entire time recommended, since the thrush may recur if the medication is stopped when the symptoms disappear.

Comfort Measures during Treatment

When treatment for thrush is started, the symptoms may seem worse for a day or two before they improve. To help speed relief, try rinsing the nipples with clear water and air drying them after each nursing, as thrush thrives on milk and moisture. Acetaminophen (Tylenol) can be safely used by the mother for pain relief.

Before the pain is gone, the following suggestions may help make nursing more comfortable:

- Offer short, frequent feedings.

- Nurse first on the less sore side (if there is one).

- Break the baby's suction before taking him off the breast by gently pulling on the baby's chin or by inserting your finger into the corner of his mouth.

Preventing Recurrence

Thrush can be harbored in many places, including milk. Once thrush has been confirmed, the following precautions may help prevent recurrence:

- Wash your hands often, especially after diaper changes and after using the toilet.

- Expressed milk can be fed to the baby, but milk expressed during a thrush outbreak should not be saved and frozen. Freezing deactivates yeast but does not kill it (Rosa 1990), so if the frozen milk is given to the baby after treatment is completed, it could cause the thrush to recur.

- If the baby uses pacifiers, bottle nipples, or teethers, boil them once a day for twenty minutes to kill the thrush. After one week of treatment, discard them and buy new ones.

- If a breast pump is used, daily boil all parts that touch the milk (except rubber gaskets).

- Disposable nursing pads should be discarded after each feeding. Cloth nursing pads should be changed after each feeding and not used again until they've been washed in hot, soapy water.

- If the baby is old enough to play with toys, anything the baby puts into his mouth should be washed frequently with hot, soapy water so that he does not re-infect himself or spread thrush to other children.

- Add *Lactobacillus acidophilus* to your diet to re-colonize your digestive tract with the good bacteria that can keep yeast in check.

- Consider eliminating sugar, yeast-containing foods and supplements, and other highly processed foods from your diet. The yeast won't have anything to feed on and you may find yourself healthier and more disease resistant in general.

Also, men can have thrush without symptoms. Thrush can be passed back and forth between husband and wife during sexual relations. If thrush continues to recur after mother and baby have had two full courses of treatment, all members of the family may need to be treated simultaneously.

References

1. Danforth D: Could it be thrush? *Leaven* 1990;26:56.

2. La Leche League International: *The Womanly Art of Breastfeeding*, 35th Anniversary Edition, Franklin Park, Illinois, La Leche League International, 1991, p.126.

3. Lawrence, R: *Breastfeeding: A Guide for the Medical Profession*, ed 3, St. Louis, Mosby, 1989, pp 392–93.

4. Mohrbacher N and Stock J: *The Breastfeeding Answer Book*, Franklin Park, Illinois, La Leche League International, 1991,pp 148–49, 172–74, 262, 429.

5. Rosa C et al: Yeasts from human milk collected in Rio de Janeiro, Brazil. *Rev Microbiol* 1990;21(4):361–63.

Chapter 39

Nursing Strikes

My Baby Is Suddenly Refusing to Nurse—Does That Mean It's Time to Wean?

A baby who is truly ready to wean will almost always do so gradually, over a period of weeks or months. If your baby or toddler has been breastfeeding well and suddenly refuses to nurse, it is probably what is called a "nursing strike" rather than a signal that it's time to wean. Nursing strikes can be frightening and upsetting to both you and your baby, but they are almost always temporary. Most nursing strikes are over, with the baby back to breastfeeding, within two to four days.

Nursing strikes happen for many reasons. They are almost always a temporary reaction to an external factor, although sometimes their cause is never determined. Here are some of the most common triggers of nursing strikes:

- You've changed your deodorant, soap, perfume, lotion, etc. and you smell "different" to your baby.

- You've been under stress (such as having extra company, traveling, moving, or dealing with a family crisis).

- Your baby or toddler has an illness or injury that makes nursing uncomfortable (an ear infection, a stuffy nose, thrush, or a cut in the mouth).

"FAQ on Nursing Strikes," last modified 1999. ©1999 La Leche League International (LLLI), www.lalecheleague.org. Reprinted with permission.

- Your baby has sore gums from teething.

- You've recently changed your nursing patterns (started a new job, left the baby with a sitter more than usual, put off nursing because of being busy, etc.).

- You reacted strongly when your baby bit you, and the baby was frightened.

Getting over the nursing strike and getting your baby back to the breast takes patience and persistence. Get medical attention if an illness or injury seems to have caused the strike. See if you can get some extra help with your household chores and older children so that you can spent lots of time with the baby. Try to relax and concentrate on making breastfeeding a pleasant experience. Stop and comfort your baby if he or she gets upset when you try to nurse. Remember that your baby isn't rejecting you, and that breastfeeding will almost always get back to normal with a little time.

Extra cuddling, stroking, and skin-to-skin contact with the baby can help you re-establish closeness. Some babies are more willing to nurse when they are sleepy. Sometimes it helps if you are rocking or walking around (in which case a sling or cloth carrier can be useful.) Try nursing in a quiet room with the lights dimmed to avoid distractions. You can also try to stimulate your let-down and get your milk flowing before offering the breast so the baby gets an immediate reward.

You will probably need to express your milk to avoid feeling uncomfortably full. You can feed the baby your milk with a cup, eye dropper, feeding syringe, or spoon. Avoid bottles; they can cause nipple confusion.

Your local LLL (La Leche League) Leader can offer support and more suggestions if these don't seem to be working.

Chapter 40

Professional Lactation Services

Chapter Contents

Section 40.1

When to Call a Lactation Professional

Information provided by the Family Collection, S. Miami Professional
Building, 7575 SW 62 Ave., Suite A, South Miami, FL 33143. Updated August
1995. Reviewed by David A. Cooke, M.D. September 29, 2001.

Before the Baby Is Born

You should call a lactation consultant for help if:

- You have flat or inverted nipples.
- You tried to nurse before but had problems.

After the Baby Is Born

You should call a lactation consultant for help if:

- The baby is not latching on or is not nursing well within forty-eight to seventy-two hours.
- You are engorged or having nipple pain longer than forty-eight hours. Breastfeeding is NOT supposed to HURT!
- You have two bad feeds in a row.
- After the third day, your baby is not having at least TWO yellow bowel movements in each twenty-four hour period.
- Your baby is sleepy and hard to wake up, or the feedings are less than eight times in a twenty-four hour period.
- You feel that your milk supply is low.
- Your baby is not gaining weight or is a slow weight gainer.
- You have plugged ducts or red area on your breast.
- You intend to return to work or school.

Section 40.2

How to Find a Lactation Professional

Women and health professionals often assume that breastfeeding is such a natural process that anyone should be able to do it without difficulty. The fact is that many women are not confident about their ability and often stop nursing their babies before they had planned due to problems that are avoidable or easily managed.

Lactation support services—both before and after the baby is born—offer information, support, and technical assistance. The following information is meant as a guide to those services.

Breastfeeding Classes

Prenatal breastfeeding classes can provide general information on breastfeeding basics, teach techniques to make it easier, and suggest problem solving strategies. Knowing the normal course of breastfeeding and how to avoid the most common pitfalls before the baby is born contributes to a longer, more satisfying breastfeeding experience. The increased knowledge and confidence is worth the few hours invested in a prenatal class.

Classes may be offered as part of a childbirth preparation series, as a separate class at a hospital, or be taught privately by a lactation professional. Sometimes a class taught by an employee of a hospital or medical group has its class content (particularly consumer issues) influenced by the employer. A good way to tell if the teacher is an employee is by whom you pay for the class. Independent practitioners usually get paid directly.

Classes are usually more effective when taught in small groups. It is desirable to have your support person attend with you. Additional features may include live demonstration of techniques and postpartum follow up by phone or personal consult. You can use the directory within or ask your childbirth educator, hospital, or health care provider for a referral.

In the event that no breastfeeding classes are available, helpful support and information can be found in a good breastfeeding book, from other nursing mothers, and by visiting breastfeeding resources on the Internet. Mother-to-mother support groups like La Leche League are also good resources.

Breast Pump Rentals

Breast pumps and other breastfeeding accessories may be rented and/or sold by rental stations. They may be individuals with or without special knowledge about breastfeeding. Types of equipment and fees vary so shop around. Some insurance policies will cover rental costs if there is a medical indication.

Lactation Professionals

Finding and choosing a lactation professional can be a confusing matter. There is a wide array of individuals who offer lactation services with different levels of training and skills. Some are licensed health practitioners while others have no medical background.

Since the field is not a licensed profession, individual practitioners may call themselves Lactation Educator, Lactation Consultant, Lactation Specialist, Lactation Counselor and so on. To find a competent practitioner you can work with, consider the criteria below.

Academic Credentials

What are their academic credentials related to breastfeeding? Where did they get their training? A practitioner may have no formal training, may have taken a university certification course, may have passed a written certification exam, or taken a correspondence course. They may be a doctor (MD), nurse (RN, LVN), occupational or physical therapist (OT, PT), a registered dietitian (RD), or speech therapist. They may call themselves a certified lactation educator (CLE), certified lactation consultant (CLC or IBCLC), a certified lactation specialist (CLS), or a certified lactation counselor (**CLC). This can be very confusing. You can ask to see their official credentials if you wish.

Experience

What did their lactation training consist of? Was there a clinical component? How many years of experience do they have? Training and experience vary widely among practitioners, so ask about it.

Services

What kind of services do they offer? Classes, phone counseling, in-person consults, rental or sales of breast pumps and other breastfeeding accessories are possibilities.

Location

Where are services provided? Are home or hospital visits made?

Fees

What are the fees for the various levels of service? Costs may be eligible for insurance reimbursement. Fee schedules vary so shop around. Some practitioners offer a sliding scale. Ask for an official bill to submit to your insurance carrier.

Business Hours

When are services available? Is there coverage for evenings and weekends?

Affiliations

Is the practitioner affiliated with a hospital or particular medical group?

Continuing Education

How does the practitioner keep up with the current research and issues in breastfeeding?

Professional Organization

Is the practitioner currently a member of a professional lactation organization?

Getting Insurance Reimbursement

In most instances, you will be asked to pay the provider of breastfeeding services directly at the time the service is given. It is the patient's responsibility to file for insurance benefits.

Not all insurance providers reimburse for breastfeeding services. They are more likely to do so if there is a medical need on the part of the mother or infant. A doctor's prescription for the service is advisable. If the medical need is for the infant (hospitalized, allergic, or premature), apply for payment on the baby's insurance claim. If the medical need is for the mother (hospitalized, breast infection), apply for payment on the mother's insurance claim. A mother returning to work and pumping her milk is not usually considered medical need.

Ask the breastfeeding service provider to give you a detailed bill complete with the corresponding insurance code numbers. Attach the doctor's prescription to the insurance form. This is more likely to make it through the system.

If your claim is denied, call the case manager and explain why the service or equipment was necessary. You may need to educate the insurance company as to the health benefits of breastfeeding and how it will save them health care costs for both the infant and mother. Make the insurance provider aware that the American Academy of Pediatrics passed a resolution recommending that third party payers provide or reimburse for lactation services as a cost effective measure.

Submitting your claim several times, each time with fuller explanations, has been known to work so keep on trying. It is helpful to explore your insurance provider's policy towards breastfeeding services before the need arises.

Section 40.3

Guide to Lactation Credentials and Abbreviations

©1999–2000, reprinted with permission of the Breastfeeding Task Force of Greater Los Angeles; 12781 Schabarum Ave., Irwindale, CA 91706; Telephone: 626-856-6650; website: www.BreastfeedingTaskForLA.org.

Abbreviations

B.A./B.S./B.S.N. Bachelor of Arts/ Science/ Nursing

C.C.E. Certified Childbirth Educator

C.L.E. Certified Lactation Educator

C.L.C. Certified Lactation Consultant

**C.L.C. Certified Lactation Counselor

C.N.S. Certified Nutrition Specialist

C.N.M. Certified Nurse Midwife

C.P.N.P. Certified Pediatric Nurse Practitioner

F.A.A.P. Fellow of American Academy of Pediatrics

H.C.C.E. Harris Certified Childbirth Educator

I.C.C.E. ICEA [International Childbirth Education Association, Inc.] Certified Childbirth Educator

I.B.C.L.C. International Board Certified Lactation Consultant

L.C.C.E. Lamaze Certified Childbirth Educator

L.V.N. Licensed Vocational Nurse

M.A. / M.S. / M.N. Master of Arts/ Science/ Nursing

M.D. Medical Doctor

M.P.H. Master of Public Health

O.T.R. Occupational Therapist Registered

R.D. Registered Dietitian

R.N.(C). Registered Nurse (Certified)

R.P.T. Registered Physical Therapist

R.R.T. Registered Respiratory Therapist

Credentials

A **Certified Lactation Educator (CLE)** has successfully completed a one week course and required homework which may include a clinical component.

A **Certified Lactation Consultant (CLC)** has had extensive formal lactation education and supervised clinical training.

An **International Board Certified Lactation Consultant (IBCLC)** has passed a certification exam and has continuing education requirements in lactation.

A **Certified Lactation Counselor (**CLC)** has taken a one week course and passed a post test.

All licensed health practitioners have additional continuing education requirements to remain current in their respective fields.

Part Six

Breastfeeding and the Working Mother

Chapter 41

Breastfeeding and Returning to Work

Why Continue to Breastfeed when Returning to Work?

- Breastmilk offers superior infant nutrition.

- Breastfed babies have significantly fewer respiratory-tract and ear infections than bottle-fed babies.

- Breastfeeding may have a long-term positive effect on an infant's immune system.

- Breastfeeding may help a mother return to her pre-pregnancy size more quickly and may lower the risk of breast cancer.

- Breastfeeding is more convenient and less expensive than bottle feeding, saving $1,000 a year in formula cost.

- Employers and communities benefit from healthier infants and children and less parent absenteeism from work.

How Does Your Employer Benefit?

- Reduced staff turnover and loss of skilled workers after the birth of a child.

This chapter includes text from: "Work and Continue to Breastfeed" © 1995 by the San Diego County Breastfeeding Coalition; reprinted with permission of San Diego County Breastfeeding Coalition, http://www.breastfeeding.org. Reviewed by David A. Cooke, M.D. September 29, 2001. And, "Breastfeeding and Returning to Work" ©1998 by Promotion of Mother's Milk (ProMoM, Inc.), www.ProMoM.com; reprinted with permission.

219

- Less sick time and personal leave due to a sick child.

- Lower and fewer health insurance claims.

- Increased job productivity, employee satisfaction, loyalty and morale.

There are several options open to mothers who wish to continue breastfeeding while working at a job that requires separation between mother and baby for several hours a day. First, and best for both

Table 41.1. Sample Letter to an Employer Requesting Accommodations for Nursing Mothers

Dear [Human Resources Manager],

This is a letter to express what I feel is an important issue and to propose what I think is a viable solution. Given the number of women who work here of childbearing age and the lack of available space in the building, privacy for nursing mothers presents a problem.

Currently, there is no facility in the building appropriate for women who need to pump breast milk. Prior to the critical space problems, women used empty offices and put out "do not disturb" signs. Currently, the only alternatives for those of us without private offices are the bathrooms or locker rooms. These facilities are not adequate or appropriate for this purpose for the following reasons:

- Unsanitary conditions (this is food for a newborn).

- Lack of privacy (pumping is a very personal and sometimes difficult process; quiet and privacy are absolutely necessary).

- Feasibility (you need somewhere to set up a pump, something to hold collection bottles, a surface on which to package the milk, and a place to sit).

I propose that the company set aside one office with several private areas partitioned off to be used by nursing mothers. This will provide not only the obvious benefits to the new mother and the new baby, but some distinct benefits to the company:

- A breastfed baby is a healthier baby. Healthier babies mean fewer medical expenses, which is a tremendous financial incentive for a self-insured company. In addition, a healthier baby means less stay-at-home days for mom.

mother and baby, is for the baby's day care provider to be located close enough to the mother's workplace for her to breastfeed the baby directly during regularly scheduled breaks. More and more firms are providing on–site or nearby day care, and are finding that the benefits for employee morale and retention make the investment worthwhile.

Second, a mother can use her break times to express her milk and bring it to the day care provider for feeding the following day. If a mother chooses this option, she will need either to learn hand-

Table 41.1. Sample Letter to an Employer Requesting Accommodations for Nursing Mothers (continued)

- An employee with fewer concerns for the welfare of her child is more able to fully focus on her job.

An employee with a convenient, sanitary, and private location for pumping will have more options in scheduling her day (for example, not having to take long lunches to drive home).

To set up a basic facility, the following things would be needed:

- A small room with a lock on the door and several keys to issue to those using the room.
- Partitions or curtains to make 2 or 3 privacy areas
- A chair and table for each privacy area.

In addition, it would be helpful to have a small sink and refrigerator in the room, as well as an electrical outlet in each privacy area.

I hope that you will consider my proposal and see what a valuable contribution this small change can make in the quality of life for a significant number of our employees. I estimate that there are probably 3 nursing women in the building at almost all times. Another company in this area has set up an excellent facility for nursing mothers and is leading a trend in corporate America. [Additional examples here.] I would like to see our company stay on the cutting edge of providing a healthy work environment and excellent benefits for employees. I believe this would be a step in that direction.

Please let me know if you have any questions or if this proposal is more appropriately directed to our site management or facilities department. I look forward to hearing from you.

Sincerely, [employee's name here]

expression technique or to rent or buy a good quality double pump. She will also need a few minutes of privacy two to three times a day. If refrigeration is not available at the workplace, storage in a cooler with "blue ice" is sufficient to preserve the milk until it can be refrigerated in the evening.

Third, a mother can breastfeed her baby when they are together and use formula when they are separated. Most mothers who try this find that their breasts quickly adjust to the daily separation, and that they have a sufficient supply for the evenings and weekends if the baby is allowed frequent access to their breasts when they are together.

Some employers may need to educated about the benefits of breastfeeding. Medela, a company that makes high-quality breast pumps, has an educational packet setting forth the cost savings to employers if their employees breastfeed their babies.

Many women are pleased and surprised to find their employers very accommodating in providing a place and time to pump or feed a baby. Often, the only reason there is no explicit policy permitting pumping or breastfeeding during work breaks is because no one has yet asked. And don't forget that in some states (Florida and Texas are in the lead on this), state law encourages employers to accommodate the needs of their employees who are breastfeeding. See Table 41.1 for a sample letter, written to the human resources manager at a large work site, which worked. The employee's need for a private and clean place to pump was accommodated.

Helpful Hints for Breastfeeding and Working

- Nurse exclusively to establish a good supply of milk before returning to work.

- At about four to six weeks, after your milk is well established and your baby is nursing well, introduce a bottle of your pumped breastmilk. Some babies are more receptive to a bottle if it is offered by someone other than you since babies usually associate breastfeeding with Mom.

- Purchase or rent a high-quality, automatic, electric breast pump.

- Familiarize yourself with the use of your electric breast pump before returning to work. Begin your pumping schedule about one to two weeks before you return.

- Use a double-pumping kit with your electric breast pump to reduce the amount of time needed to express your milk. Most mothers can complete a pumping session in 10 to 15 minutes by expressing both breasts simultaneously.

- To ease your transition back to work, try to return midweek so that you have only a few days before the weekend.

- If your company does not have a special room for mothers who are breastpumping, find a spot that is as private and comfortable as possible. Bring something to drink, a small snack, and a picture of your baby to make your surroundings feel more like home. If you have difficulty letting down, take a few deep breaths, listen to soothing music, and look at a picture of your baby.

- Select a supportive caregiver for your baby.

- Give your caregiver explicit written instructions on how to store, thaw, and warm breastmilk.

- Explain to your caregiver that, if possible, your baby should not be fed within a couple of hours of your return, so your baby will be ready to breastfeed as soon as you come home from work.

Tips for Success

- Give yourself and your family time to settle in to your new life.

- Drink plenty of fluids and eat a nutritious diet of wholesome foods.

- Ask family members or friends to help with meals and housework. Focus on the things that really need to be accomplished.

- Give yourself time to rest when you get home from work.

- Ask other family members to cuddle and comfort the baby while you do other tasks.

- Prepare your baby's father for his role in supporting your breastfeeding activities.

- Consult a lactation professional for information and support.

Talk with Your Employer before Your Baby Is Born

- Explain to your employer the health benefits of breastfeeding for your baby.

- Let your employer know that less absenteeism among breastfeeding mothers is a bonus for cost-conscious employers.

- Discuss your company's maternity leave, part time work and job sharing policies and arrange for flexible breaks and work hours to accommodate pumping and breastfeeding.

- Encourage your employer to provide a private area that is clean and comfortable to express milk during work hours and a small refrigerator for safe storage of breastmilk.

These are some ideas about how to go about breastfeeding after returning to work. If you have any other questions, contact La Leche League International or a lactation professional. to obtain additional information about such issues as hand expressing human milk, obtaining and using breast pumps, storing and using expressed breastmilk, and other questions pertaining to working and breastfeeding.

Chapter 42

How to Choose a Breastpump

Find One That's Right for You

There are several types of breastpumps on the market today made by a variety of companies. The choices can be overwhelming. See Table 42.1 for help in choosing the best breastpump for your situation. Also, consider the following when shopping for a breastpump.

Why will be using this pump? Do you plan to use a pump to establish your milk supply, increase your milk supply, feed a premature baby, or provide an occasional supplement when you may be away from your baby during a feeding time? Some pumps are better at establishing a milk supply then others.

How frequently do you plan to use the pump? Will you be pumping one or twice a week or several times a day? If you do not plan on pumping too frequently, you may want to consider hand expressing or using a hand pump. If you plan on pumping often, you may want to consider a semi-automatic or self-cycling electric pump.

Do you plan to pump on one side while your baby nurses on the other? If this is the case, you'll want a pump that can be easily operated with one hand. For this situation, consider a squeeze-handle hand pump, a battery-operated pump, or a semi-automatic electric pump.

Do you plan to pump at least once a day? Then you may want to consider an automatic self-cycling electric pump.

Other things to consider when shopping for a pump include how easy it is to use and if it comes with an adapter for the cigarette lighter in your car—something handy and sometimes essential for pumping in your car!

You may also want to consider a pump that is easy to carry and store. Having two breastpump kits (the breast shield, valve, piston, cylinder, and other parts that are detachable from the pump itself) can come in handy. Many women will leave one kit and at home and take the other to work.

The basic types of breastpumps are manual hand pumps, battery-operated pumps, semi-automatic electric pumps, and self-cycling electric pumps.

While electric pumps are more efficient than hand or battery-operated pumps, they are also more expensive to buy. However, often times these pumps can be rented. Other advantages to electric pumps is that most of these pumps are well serviced by the manufacturers and in some circumstances, may be covered by health insurance.

Battery-operated pumps are best for women who have an established milk supply and want to pump a little once or twice a day or less. Some disadvantages include that they are not adequate to stimulate production and the baby often has to be feeding while pumping to stimulate the breast.

While most hand pumps are inexpensive and portable, some are difficult to clean and can sometimes cause trauma to the breast.

Table 42.1. Choosing the Best Breastpump for Your Situation

If You Want To:	Then the Best Pump Is:
Establish milk supply	Self-cycling electric pump
Increase milk supply	Any pump on the market or hand expressing
Pump an occasional supplement	Hand pump, battery-operated pump, semi-automatic electric pump, or hand expressing
Pump for a hospitalized preemie	Self-cycling electric pump
Pump1–2 times per week	Hand pump, battery-operated pump, semi-automatic electric pump, or hand expressing
Pump at least once a day	Semi-automatic electric or self-cycling electric pump
Pump on one side while baby nurses on other	Battery-operated pump, semi-automatic electric pump, or self-cycling electric pump
Double pump	Semi-automatic electric or self-cycling electric pump

Chapter 43

Tips for Successful Pumping

- Pump at approximately the same time each day.

- If separated from your baby, pump at the times your baby usually feeds.

- Promoting the milk-ejection reflex (let-down) with a relaxed environment, warm compresses, and gentle breast massage will improve milk flow.

- When single pumping, move the breast cup back and forth between breasts several times throughout the pumping session to improve milk yield.

- Don't be discouraged if your first attempts result in very little milk yield. Regular pumping usually results in ample yield in one to two weeks.

- Store milk in amounts baby is expected to consume in a single feeding to avoid waste.

- Milk may be stored in glass or rigid plastic baby bottles. Label bottle with date, time of collection, and any unusual food or medicine consumed. Milk may be refrigerated for use within forty-eight and seventy-two hours. Freezing is recommended for

©1999–2000, reprinted with permission of the Breastfeeding Task Force of Greater Los Angeles; 12781 Schabarum Ave., Irwindale, CA 91706; Telephone: 626-856-6650; website: www.BreastfeedingTaskForLA.org.

later use. Acceptable times for frozen storage vary with the temperature of the freezer. (See Chapter 44, Concerns when Storing Human Milk, for more information about storing breastmilk.)

- Raw human milk separates on standing with fat rising to the top. Just shake gently to redistribute fat particles evenly.

- Human milk should be gently warmed to body temperature by standing the bottle in a bowl of warm water. Heating in boiling water or a microwave may destroy some components in human milk and scald your baby during a feeding.

- Your baby may resist initial attempts to take milk in a bottle. Using a newborn-size, slow flow nipple, and having someone else offer the feeding may make it easier. Depending on the age of the baby, cup or spoon feeding may be more acceptable. BE PATIENT!

- If you require assistance, please seek help from a lactation professional or your local La Leche League. (See Chapter 40, Professional Lactation Services, for help in locating a lactation professional.)

Chapter 44

Concerns when Storing Human Milk

One of the many benefits of breastfeeding is convenience. Most of the time, human milk goes directly from producer to consumer, with no concerns about collection, storage, preparation, or freshness in between. However, some mothers express and save milk for their babies, either occasionally or regularly. This article addresses some common questions and concerns about the appearance of expressed milk and safe storage of human milk for healthy, full-term babies. If your baby is hospitalized or you are collecting milk for a milk bank, different guidelines may apply.

Visual Characteristics of Human Milk

Those who have never seen human milk may be surprised if they expect it to look like cow's milk out of a carton. Unlike homogenized milk, human milk will separate when left to stand, with the fat rising to the top. This does not mean it has spoiled. Simply shaking the container gently will restore the milk to a homogeneous consistency.

Samples of human milk expressed at different times may not look the same either, as various factors can influence fat content and even color. The amount of fat can fluctuate from day to day and within a nursing or pumping session as well. Milk expressed at the

From "Common Concerns When Storing Human Milk," by Cindy Scott Duke, *New Beginnings*, July-August 1998. Reprinted with permission from La Leche League International (LLLI), www.lalecheleague.org.

beginning of a feeding may look "thinner" than milk expressed later, when the milk-ejection reflex sends milk higher in fat toward the nipple.

The color of human milk can vary. Colostrum is generally yellow to yellow-orange. The transition from colostrum to mature milk can take about two weeks to complete. During that time, the color changes gradually to a bluish white color. However, the color of mature milk may change because of mother's diet or medications. Food dyes used in carbonated sodas, fruit drinks, and gelatin desserts have been associated with milk that is pink or pinkish-orange. Greenish milk has been linked to consuming green-colored sports beverages, seaweed, or large amounts of green vegetables. One woman consuming a certain prescription medication reported black milk. Frozen milk may look yellowish.

Pinkish milk may indicate blood in the milk. This could occur with or without cracked nipples. If cracked nipples are the cause of blood in the milk, a mother can contact a La Leche League Leader for suggestions on healing sore nipples. Blood in milk is not harmful to babies, and breastfeeding can continue. If blood in the milk does not cease by two weeks postpartum, the mother may wish to consult with her health care provider.

Odor of Human Milk

Under most circumstances, fresh human milk has a mild, slightly sweet scent. Occasionally, human milk that has been frozen and thawed may smell soapy and may be rejected by the baby. In *Breastfeeding: A Guide for the Medical Profession*, Ruth Lawrence, MD, postulates that for some mothers, milk stored in a self-defrosting freezer may have had changes in its lipid structure due to the freeze-thaw cycles that occur in such freezers.

In a few cases, mothers have reported that their milk began to smell soapy as soon as it cooled, regardless of whether it had been frozen. "When these mothers heated their milk to a scald (not boiling) and then quickly cooled and froze it," writes Lawrence, "the effect was not apparent and their infants accepted the heat treated milk. That process inactivated the lipase (fat-digesting enzyme) and halted the process of fat digestion." However, high heating may lower some nutrient levels, including ascorbic acid (vitamin C). If the milk already smells sour, heating will have no effect on flavor or smell. Milk that smells rancid likely is, and should be discarded.

Choosing a Milk Storage Container

After expressing milk into a clean container, milk should be stored in a tightly closed glass or plastic container. There have been controversies about what type of container will best protect the nutrients and immunity factors in human milk. Current research suggests that human milk can safely be stored in glass or plastic receptacles with no significant nutrient loss. *The Breastfeeding Answer Book* recommends glass, clear hard plastic (polycarbonate), and cloudy hard plastic (polypropylene)—in that order—as storage containers for freezing milk. If a baby receives expressed milk only occasionally, any possible effect of the container on the quality of the milk will be negligible.

Ease of use can be an important consideration when choosing a container. Plastic bags take up less room and can be connected directly to some breast pumps. Bags designed specifically for storing human milk are constructed of thicker material, are easily sealable, presterilized, and have space to label the milk with the date and baby's name. Disposable polyethylene bottle liners are not designed to store milk and are not recommended. The seams may burst during freezing, and the bag can leak during thawing. If you must use these, double bagging can help avoid tearing. These bags are not recommended for long-term storage.

Cooled milk can be combined with other cooled or frozen milk as long as the quantity of cooled milk is small enough that it doesn't thaw a frozen batch. Freezing milk in small quantities (2 to 4 oz. or 60–120 ml.) helps avoid wasting this precious fluid. Label with the date and your baby's name if it will be stored with milk for more than one baby.

Short-Term Storage when Refrigeration Is Not Available

Lack of immediate access to refrigeration need not be a deterrent to expressing and storing human milk or dampen a mother's determination to continue breastfeeding if she returns to work. Research shows that human milk has an amazing capacity to resist bacterial growth, and can be kept at room temperature for up to ten hours. In a landmark study, mature human milk was expressed into clean (not sterile) containers, some stored at room temperature (19–22° C or 66 to 72° F) and some refrigerated for ten hours. The milk was then cultured to evaluate bacterial formation. No statistically significant difference was found between levels of bacteria in the milk that had been refrigerated and the milk stored at room temperature (Barger and Bull 1987).

Small coolers (some designed especially for human milk) and wide-mouthed insulated bottles can be used to keep milk cool when electric refrigeration is unavailable. An insulated bottle can be filled with ice before leaving the house to keep the interior chilled. The ice should be emptied just before pouring expressed milk into the bottle.

How long will the milk be good? Storage guidelines based on current research are below. If your milk will be fed to your baby by someone other than you, you may find it helpful to provide them with a copy of the guidelines.

Milk to be used within eight days of expression should be refrigerated rather than frozen. Not only will the milk not need to be thawed, but the immunity factors in human milk are better preserved by refrigeration. For longer storage, milk can be frozen.

Keep in mind that the composition of the mother's milk corresponds to the developmental needs of her baby at the time the milk was produced, and try to use the freshest milk possible.

Storing Milk Away from Home

A lactating mother should face no restrictions storing her milk somewhere other than her own home, such as a workplace or day care refrigerator. No special precautions apply. If an employed mother does encounter resistance from coworkers, it may be lessened if the milk is placed in an opaque, secondary container, suggests Laurie Nommsen-Rivers in the *Journal of Human Lactation* (1997). There are several sources of information a mother can use to educate others not only about the benefits of human milk but to alleviate any concerns they may have about safe storage of a "body fluid."

In an October 1995 press release, the Center for Breastfeeding Information at La Leche League International stated, "As of this date, human milk is not (nor has it ever been) included in federal health agencies' listings of body fluids governed by universal precautions for blood-borne pathogens which would mandate handling and feeding with rubber gloves or storage in a separate refrigerator as a biohazardous material. This continues to be the current policy of the United States Centers for Disease Control and Prevention (CDC) and the Occupational Safety and Health Administration (OSHA)." Other countries have considered the idea of universal precautions, however, "specifics regarding breastmilk are hard to find," according to Nommsen-Rivers.

Caring for Our Children, a 1992 joint publication by the American Academy of Pediatrics and the American Public Health Association (with input from the Human Milk Banking Association of North America), offers guidelines for out-of-home child care programs. This work recognizes, supports, and promotes the feeding of human milk to infants in day care and places no restrictions beyond regular hand washing and standard refrigeration protocols. *Caring for Our Children* is available from: AAP Publications Dept, P.0. Box 927, Elk Grove Village IL 60009-0927. Phone: 800-433-9016; FAX: 708-228-1281.

Mothers who are separated from their babies may have many other questions and concerns beyond milk storage, including easing separation for both mother and baby, pumps and pumping, manual (hand) expression, or making a return to work easier. La Leche League Leaders can be valuable resources for these considerations.

Human Milk Storage Information

This information is based on current research and applies to mothers who:

- have healthy full-term babies,

- are storing their milk for home use (as opposed to hospital use),

- wash their hands before expressing, and

- use containers that have been washed in hot, soapy water and rinsed.

All milk should be dated before storing.

Storage Guidelines

Term Colostrum (expressed within six days of delivery)

- can be kept at room temperature 27–32 C (80.6–89.6° F) for 12 hours

Mature Milk

- can be stored at 15 C (59–60° F) for 24 hours

- can be stored at 19–22 C (66–72° F) for 10 hours

- can be stored at 25 C (79° F) for 4–6 hours

- can be refrigerated at 0–4 C (32–39° F) for 8 days

Frozen Milk

- can be stored in a freezer compartment located inside a refrigerator for 2 weeks

- can be stored in a separate door refrigerator/freezer for 3 or 4 months (temperature varies because the door opens frequently)

- can be stored in a separate deep freeze at constant -19 C (0° F) for 6 months or longer

What Type of Containers to Use for Freezing Milk

- heavy plastic or glass containers can be used

- freezer milk bags are available that are designed for storing human milk

- disposable bottle liners are not recommended

- cool milk in refrigerator before adding to a container of frozen milk.

How to Warm the Milk

Thaw and/or heat under warm running water, but do not bring temperature of milk to boiling point. Shake before testing the temperature, and never use a microwave oven to heat human milk.

If milk has been frozen and thawed, it can be refrigerated up to 24 hours for later use. It should not be refrozen.

References

1. Barger J and Bull P: A comparison of the bacterial composition of breast milk stored at room temperature and stored in the refrigerator. *Intl J Childbirth Ed* 1987;2:29–30.

2. Nommsen-Rivers L: Universal precautions are not needed for health care workers handling breast milk. *J Hum Lact* 1997;13(4):267–68.

Part Seven

Special Situations

Chapter 45

Breastfeeding after a Cesarean Section

Studies show that women whose babies are born by cesarean surgery are just as successful at breastfeeding as mothers who deliver vaginally, as long as their commitment to breastfeeding remains high. It may, however, take a bit longer for mothers and babies to begin breastfeeding after cesarean surgery, and mothers' milk tends to come in a bit later following a surgical birth. This may be a direct result of the surgery, or it may be because mothers who have cesareans have fewer opportunities for early and frequent breastfeeding.

If you know before you go into labor that you will be having a cesarean, talk to your doctor ahead of time about holding and nursing your baby immediately after the birth. Even if your cesarean was not the birth you anticipated, you can still make the most of the your baby's first feedings. You will need extra help, since you're doing double duty: healing yourself and feeding your baby. Following are some time-tested helpers for successfully breastfeeding following a surgical birth.

Ask to see and hold your baby as soon as possible after birth. With help from nurses and your partner, you can enjoy skin-to-skin contact and give your baby an opportunity to nuzzle at your breast.

"Breastfeeding after a Cesarean," at www.askdrsears.com, 2000, by Dr. William P. Sears © AskDrSears.com. Used with permission. Information about Dr. Sears can be found at the end of this chapter or at www.askdrsears.com.

Plan to breastfeed your baby in the recovery room before the anesthesia wears off. With help from nurses, or your partner, you can put baby to the breast even if you must lie flat in bed.

Your doctor can prescribe pain medication for you that will not affect your baby. Pain suppresses milk production and makes it harder for you to enjoy your newborn. To decrease postoperative pain, talk to your anesthesiologist about using medications that will help you feel the most comfortable, yet alert, after the surgery. Long-acting analgesics (for example, Duramorph) injected into the spinal tubing immediately after birth can considerably ease postoperative pain.

Discuss with your doctor the use of "patient-controlled analgesia" (PCA) in which you administer your own pain-relieving medication as you need relief. Don't hesitate to use pain medication—you and your baby will enjoy each other more if you are comfortable.

Plan to breastfeed early and often. When baby is hungry or fussing, have one of your attendants (either the nurse or your spouse), bring baby to you and help you position his body and mouth for efficient latch-on.

Ask your lactation consultant or attending nurse to show you how to breastfeed in the side-lying and clutch-hold positions. These positions keep baby's weight off your incision. Lying down while nursing helps you rest and relax.

When nursing in the side-lying position, comfortably surround yourself with pillows. Place one or two pillows between your back and the side-rail, another pillow between your knees, a pillow under your head, and one under baby. To support your incision while lying on your side, wedge a tummy pillow (a small, foam cushion or even a folded bath towel) between the bed and your abdomen.

If you sit up in bed to nurse your baby, use lots of pillows to support your body. Put pillows under your knees to take the strain off your abdomen and back. Pillows on your lap under baby will protect your incision. You may find nursing sessions more comfortable if you get out of bed and sit in a chair.

Be sure your partner watches how the professionals help you breastfeed. Have them show him how to help you in the hospital and later on at home. It's especially important for dads to learn how to help you with the lower-lip flip.

As much as possible, keep your baby with you in your room after a cesarean. Rooming-in is possible, even after a surgical birth. Get help from dad, grandma, or a friend—someone who can be with you most of the time in the hospital and lend a hand with the baby.

The decisions and details surrounding a cesarean birth may seem overwhelming at times. Don't let this distract you from your precious time with your new baby. Do whatever you can to enjoy these first few days together.

About the Author

Dr. William Sears, M.D. is Associate Clinical Professor of Pediatrics at the University of California, Irvine, School of Medicine, and the co-author of numerous books on childbirth and parenting including *The Baby Book* (Little Brown & Co., 1992) and *The Breastfeeding Book* (Little Brown & Co., 2000). He is also a medical and parenting consultant for *BabyTalk* and *Parenting* magazines. Additional information about Dr. Sears can be found at www.askdrsears.com/aboutdrsears.asp.

Chapter 46

Breastfeeding More than One Baby

Breastfeeding more than one baby can be very special, but it also demands work and patience in the first few months. Here are answers to some common questions about nursing your babies.

Will I Have Enough Milk?

Your body works on supply and demand, so you should be able to make enough milk for more than one baby. Try to eat three balanced meals and two snacks, drink when you are thirsty, rest when you can, and take one day at a time.

You may also need to continue taking the iron and vitamin pills you took while you were pregnant.

Be sure to drink enough fluids. You will find that you are most thirsty during nursing. It is a good idea to drink enough fluids so your urine is pale yellow. Each time you feed your babies, drink one to two eight-ounce glasses of water, juice, or milk (drink some of each).

Rest whenever you can. Sleep when your babies are asleep instead of doing housework. Try to make your life as simple as you can. Do not start any projects that can be put off for a few weeks or months.

How Will I Know My Babies Are Getting Enough Milk?

Once your milk is in, your babies are getting enough milk if they each:

Patient Information Sheet 147. University Hospitals Health System, University Hospitals of Cleveland. ©1998, used with permission.

- Wet at least six cloth or five disposable diapers a day.
- Nurse eight to twelve times in twenty-four hours.
- Gain one pound a month.

How Often Do I Feed My Babies?

Feed your babies whenever they seem hungry. In the first week or two, they may seem hungry all the time. This is normal and doesn't mean you do not have enough milk. It may mean that all you do for the first weeks is feed your babies.

Life may be very busy for you until the babies settle into a routine at around two to three weeks of age. Babies also go through growth spurts some time around seven to ten days, six weeks, three months, and six months old. You may find they need to nurse constantly at these times. This also is normal and lasts only about two days.

What If the Babies Are Hungry at the Same Time?

Many mothers feed the hungry baby or babies first and then wake up the other baby or babies and feed them. But there will be times when you are faced with two or more crying, hungry babies at the same time. In this case, you can distract the baby or babies while you feed the other, or feed two at the same time. Ways to distract your baby include:

- Give your baby a pacifier.
- Place your baby in a swing, cradle, or stroller and rock it with your foot.
- Let someone else hold your baby.

There are several good basic books on breastfeeding that can be used for multiple babies as well. Ask your nurse for names or titles of the books. Below are a few more methods for feeding twins.

You may choose to have someone help with feedings. You can do this by having someone feed one baby a bottle of pumped breastmilk while you nurse the other baby or babies. Then switch at the next feeding and nurse the baby or babies who received the bottle.

If nursing one baby at a time, keep the first baby on one breast only and nurse longer. When the second baby is nursed on the other breast, you can be assured there is an ample milk supply.

When breast feeding both infants at a feeding, be sure to rotate the breast given to each baby since each baby's suck and stimulation may be different.

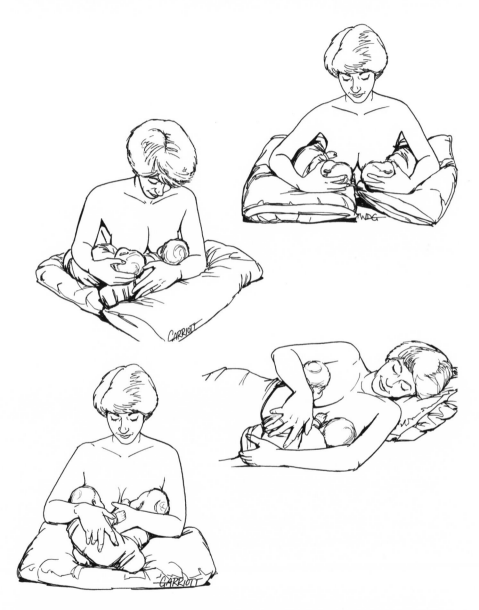

Figure 46.1. Here are some ways for you to breastfeed both of your babies at the same time.

Chapter 47

Breastfeeding the Adopted Baby

Are you are about to adopt a baby and you want to breastfeed him? Wonderful! It is not only possible, it is fairly easy and the chances are you will produce a significant amount of milk. It is not complicated, but it is different than breastfeeding a baby with whom you have been pregnant for nine months.

Breastfeeding and Breastmilk

There are really two objectives involved in nursing an adopted baby. One is getting your baby to breastfeed. The other is producing breastmilk. It is important to set your expectations at a reasonable level. Since there is more to breastfeeding than breastmilk, many mothers are happy to be able to breastfeed without expecting to produce all the milk the baby will need. It is the special relationship, the special closeness, the biological attachment of breastfeeding that many mothers are looking for. As one adopting mother said, "I want to breastfeed. If the baby also gets breastmilk, that's great."

Getting the Baby to Take the Breast

Although many people do not believe that the early introduction of bottles may interfere with breastfeeding, the early introduction of artificial nipples can indeed interfere. The sooner you can get the baby

Handout 23, "Breastfeeding Your Adopted Baby" by Jack Newman, M.D., F.R.C.P.C. Revised January 1998, reprinted with permission.

to the breast after he is born, the better. However, babies need flow from the breast in order to stay latched on and continue sucking, especially if they have gotten used to get flow from a bottle or another method of feeding (cup, finger feeding). So, what can you do?

1. Speak with the staff at the hospital where the baby will be born and let the head nurse and lactation consultant know you plan to breastfeed the baby. They should be willing to accommodate your desire to have the baby fed by cup or finger feeding if you cannot have the baby to feed immediately after his birth. In fact, more and more frequently, arrangements have been made where the adopting mother is present at the birth of the baby and takes the baby immediately to nurse. The earlier you start, the better.

2. Some biological mothers are willing to nurse the baby for the first few days. There is some concern expressed amongst social workers and others that this will result in the biological mother changing her mind. This is possible, and you may not wish to take that risk. However, this has been done, and it allows the baby to breastfeed, get colostrum, and not receive artificial feedings at first.

3. Latching on well is just as important (in fact, even more important) when the mother does not have a full milk supply as when she does. A good latch means painless feedings. A good latch means the baby will get more of your milk, whether your milk supply is abundant or minimal.

4. If the baby does need to be supplemented, this should be done with a lactation aid with the supplement being given while the baby is breastfeeding. Babies learn to breastfeed by breastfeeding, not cup feeding or finger feeding or bottle feeding. Of course, you can use your previously expressed milk to supplement.

5. If you are having trouble getting the baby to take the breast, see a lactation professional as soon as possible for help.

Producing Breastmilk

As soon as a baby is in sight, start getting your milk supply ready. Please understand, you may never produce a full supply for your baby, though it may happen. You should not be discouraged by what you may be pumping before the baby is born, because a pump is never as good at extracting milk as a baby who is sucking well and well latched. The main purpose of pumping before the baby is born is to start the changes in your breast so that you will produce milk, not to build up a reserve of milk before the baby is born (though this is good if you can do it.)

If you can manage it, rent an electric pump with a double setup. Pumping both breasts at the same time takes half the time, obviously, but also results in better milk production. Start pumping as soon as the baby is in sight, even if this means you will be pumping for 4 months. You do not have to pump frequently on a schedule. Do what is possible. If twice a day is possible at first, do twice a day. If once a day during the week, but six times during the weekend can be done, fine. Partners can help with nipple stimulation as well.

Domperidone is a drug that can help you produce more milk. It is not necessary for you to use in order to breastfeed an adopted baby, but it will help you develop a more abundant milk supply faster. There is no such thing as a 100% safe drug. If you do decide to take it, the dose is 20 mg four times a day. Ask your doctor for more information.

Using pumping and domperidone, most adopting mothers have started to produce drops of milk after two to four weeks.

Will you produce all the milk the baby needs? Maybe, but don't count on it. Some breastmilk is better than none. Even if you do not, breastfeed your baby, and allow both of you to enjoy the special relationship that it brings.

Chapter 48

Breastfeeding the Baby with Special Needs

My new baby was born with a disability. Can I still breastfeed?

If your baby was born with special challenges, you are probably struggling with conflicting feelings. Like most parents, you are joyful and excited to meet your new baby. At the same time, you may having feelings of disappointment, anger, helplessness, even guilt.

Babies born with Down syndrome, cleft lip or palate, cardiac problems, cystic fibrosis, or a neurological impairment need the benefits of breastmilk even more than other babies. The perfect nutrition and immunological benefits of human milk will keep your baby as healthy as possible, so they are better able to gain weight and be strong for any surgeries or treatment they may need. Also, the special bond and breastfeeding hormones of the breastfeeding mother will help to keep you calmer and more in touch with your baby as a person first, a challenged baby second.

Breastmilk is easily digestible and better for the health of babies with heart problems or cystic fibrosis, who may have trouble gaining weight. It is less irritating to the nasal passages of a baby with a cleft palate than artificial milk (formula) is. Breastmilk will help protect the baby with Down Syndrome from the respiratory infections and bowel problems he or she may be prone to.

"FAQ on Breastfeeding Babies with Special Needs," last modified 1999. ©1999 La Leche League International (LLLI), www.lalecheleague.org. Reprinted with permission.

Often a challenged baby is reluctant to take the breast. If you are determined to make it work, let your medical team know. Your partner, other family members and friends, your lactation consultant, and your LLL (La Leche League) Leader can back you up. If you want to give your milk to your baby, try to breastfeed right away. If this isn't working, start pumping as soon as possible after birth. You should pump as often as a baby would breastfeed, every two to three hours. The milk can be given by naso-gastric tube or some other feeding method. It's best to avoid bottles and pacifiers, because your baby has to suck differently on a bottle and may become so nipple confused that it will be harder to get him to take the breast when he's ready.

Ask your Leader or lactation consultant about getting a Supplemental Feeding System (SNS). You fill a small bottle with your milk, and a thin tube passes from it, which you tape to your breast or your finger, and feed that way. Your finger is more similar to your nipple than a rubber bottle nipple is. Some doctors and nurses are unfamiliar with this method. Tell them about why it is important to you and your baby. Keep trying to breastfeed, if at all possible. It's been proven by research that breastfeeding is less stressful for babies than bottle feeding, but your doctor may not know this.

When you are ready to attempt breastfeeding, be prepared to be patient. It may take a few weeks for your baby to learn how to properly latch on. Again, seek the support of your LLL Leader or lactation consultant. A neurologically impaired baby, with too much or too little muscle tone, may need extra kinds of support while nursing. The cuddling and skin-to-skin contact involved in breastfeeding provides the stimulation your baby needs to fully develop his capabilities.

If your doctor wants you to supplement a slow-gaining baby, see if he will agree to using your hindmilk (the milk in your breast at the end of a feeding, which has a higher fat/calorie content). You can express and give this by another feeding method if the baby is not sucking effectively. A baby with cystic fibrosis or PKU (phenylketonuria) may need extra digestive enzymes.

In some cases, the challenged baby may never become an avid breastfeeder. Rest assured that any amount of your breastmilk—received at your breast, pumped and given by bottle, or provided by some other method (SNS, syringe, spoon, naso-gastric tube, Habermann Feeder)—will greatly benefit your baby's health and development. It's something you alone can provide, which is good for your morale!

Chapter 49

Breastfeeding the Baby with a Cleft Lip or Palate

Most mothers want the best for their children, and we all agree that breastfeeding our newborn child is best. Breastfeeding ensures that baby is getting the best of all possible foods. Breastfeeding strengthens the mother-child bond. Breastfeeding is natural. And, breastfeeding offers additional protective elements that help to ensure the health and well being of our child.

When a child is born with a cleft, it is not a foregone conclusion that that child will not be able to breastfeed. If the cleft affects only the lip and alveolar ridge, there is a very good chance that the baby will eventually be able to breastfeed successfully. However, lacking an intact palate, most babies cannot form the negative pressure that is an essential ingredient to successfully latching on.

When a child is born with a birth defect—any birth defect—parents must initially grieve the loss of the perfect child they had imagined they would have. When that birth defect precludes breastfeeding, the mother suffers another loss—the loss of her imagined role as mother. At the same time, she suffers the loss of control in her life.

Because some babies with clefts—even cleft palates—do indeed feed successfully at the breast, mothers who wish to try should be

From "Breastfeeding the Cleft-Affected Newborn: Making It Safe," ©1996 available online at http://www.widesmiles.org/cleftlinks/WS-004.html; and "Cleft and Nursing: The Basic Facts," © 1997 available online at http://widesmiles.org/cleftlinks/WS-745.html. Both documents reprinted with the permission of WideSmiles, www.widesmiles.org.

251

encouraged to do so. But there are some cautions that must be seriously heeded.

Be prepared for a great deal of frustration before there will be success. Contrary to popular thought, babies are not born knowing how to breastfeed. All babies must be taught how to use their instinctive rooting and suckling responses to elicit sustenance from a breast. A cleft-affected child has those same instincts, but she does not have the same structure that would help her to use those instincts for successful feeding. You and she must experiment until you find the method that will work for you.

Know the signs of dehydration and seek medical attention at the FIRST sign of problems. Because breastfeeding may be difficult for your baby, and because many attempts may result in either little milk or no milk at all getting into baby's tummy, you must be constantly aware of possible signs and symptoms of dehydration—a potentially lethal complication of breastfeeding frustration. The signs of dehydration include a sleepy, listless baby; a baby who wets fewer than ten times per every twenty-four hours; or urine that is strong smelling, concentrated, and/or dark in color. If any of those signs are present in your baby while you are attempting to learn a breastfeeding pattern, take your child to a doctor or a hospital immediately. Also, watch your baby's weight carefully. If your baby loses more than 10% of her body weight, or more than one pound, see your doctor immediately.

Go ahead and give it a try. If you and your child succeed in breastfeeding, the rewards can be immense. But don't be too stubborn about it. After all, your primary goal should be to put nutrition into your baby's stomach that will help her to grow and stay healthy.

Accepting that your child will not be able to suckle at your breast does not mean that she cannot be sustained by your breastmilk. You may have to learn how to pump your own breasts and feed your child with a bottle.

Bottle feeding your infant will not inhibit your mother-child bond. After all, your child's father may also be closely bonded to the baby, and he cannot breastfeed her either. Make sure there is a lot of holding and cuddling going on, and hold your baby close to your body when you do feed her.

Bear in mind that while all things being equal, breastfeeding is best, all things are not always equal and there are times when a bottle is needed to ensure the well-being of your precious child. Even though we know that the breast is best, bottle feeding your infant does not constitute child abuse, and it could be the best way for YOUR child to eat.

Some Basic Facts

- A child with a cleft lip CAN and most likely WILL successfully nurse at the breast.

- The alveolar ridge does NOT determine whether a child can nurse at the breast or not.

- A child with a cleft palate does NOT possess the mechanics necessary to allow him/her to nurse at the breast.

- A child with an intact lip and/or alveolar ridge BUT a cleft palate is NOT likely to successfully nurse at the breast.

- Very few babies can nurse at the breast after palate repair.

- Lip repair will NOT facilitate nursing at the breast.

- If a child has a cleft of the soft palate, an obturator will not facilitate nursing at the breast.

Exceptions to all of the above occur, but are exceptionally rare. These exceptions are based on a combination of the unique character of each individual cleft and of a mother's ability to let down, the size of the breast tissue, etc.

As much as we would like to think otherwise, doctors, nurses, and even lactation consultants may not know about breastfeeding a child with a cleft. Their degree and/or certification does not necessarily prepare them for the unique challenges of nursing a cleft-affected child at the breast. In all cases, each mother/ child team must learn what they can and cannot accomplish. Nursing at the breast may be a family's first choice, but it is not their only choice.

Chapter 50

Breastfeeding the Premature Baby

Is Breastfeeding Important for My Premature Baby?

Tiny, pre-term babies need their mother's good milk even more than full-term babies. If your baby was born earlier than expected, you are probably awash in a storm of feelings. Feelings of protectiveness come over you when you see his tiny, frail-looking body. You may be feeling afraid, angry, or guilty. The busy, bustling medical team may be making you feel out of place, like you're not really needed, not even a real parent!

But you are needed, and in a big way. The milk from your breasts is something you alone can provide for your baby. It contains invaluable nutrients and immune properties that can make a big difference in the health of your baby and in his development. The milk produced by the mother of a pre-term infant is higher in protein and other nutrients than the milk produced by the mother of a term infant. Human milk also contains lipase, an enzyme which allows the baby to digest fat more efficiently. Your breastfed preemie is less likely to develop infections that plague artificially fed babies. He will be protected by the immune properties in your milk while his own immature immune system is developing.

Your fresh milk is best for your baby. Donor milk must be pasteurized, which kills its infection-fighting live cells (though is certainly a good alternative when a mother is unable to provide her own milk).

Providing your milk, either directly at the breast or by pumping, benefits you and baby in other ways. The loving bond you feel as the milk flows is good for your relationship. It helps you to think of your baby as a person first, your very own beloved child, and not just the doctor's medical case. This bond will sustain both of you through any difficulties that lie ahead.

How Do I Breastfeed My Pre-Term Baby?

Perhaps your baby is strong and mature enough to feed directly at your breast. It may take some time to encourage him to do it correctly. Try the cross cradle hold. This allows you to get a better view of the baby, and to control the baby's head. Position the baby across your lap, turned in towards you, chest to chest. Use pillows to bring him up to the level of your breast. If you are offering your right breast, hold the baby's head in your left hand, and support your breast with your right. Your baby may need help to open his mouth wide enough. Ask a nurse or relative to help by pressing gently down on the baby's chin.

Research has found that breastfeeding is less stressful than bottle feeding for babies, so let your doctor know you prefer to put the baby to the breast when he is ready, instead of bottle feeding. To encourage a reluctant baby, you may want to try a Supplemental Feeding System on your nipple or finger. Your LLL (La Leche League) Leader or lactation consultant will be able to get you one.

What about Pumping My Milk?

If your baby is not strong enough to feed at the breast, you should begin to pump as soon after the birth as you are able. Frequent pumping, every two to three hours, will mimic the frequency of a newborn's feeding pattern, and bring in a good milk supply. Get a full-size, hospital-grade pump with a double-pump kit. Doing both breasts at once will save you time. Save your colostrum, the first milk. This is the perfect first feed for your baby to have.

What Is Kangaroo Care?

A practice gaining in popularity, since it has been shown to be beneficial to babies, is called "kangaroo care." When your baby is strong enough to come out of the isolette, hold him, skin-to-skin, on your chest. Your warmth, smell, and familiar heartbeat will feel like a warm womb with a view to your baby. He will be soothed and calmed. This will aid in his development. He may start to root for your breast and try to nurse for the first time. Fathers can carry their babies this way too, and feel connected.

As much as you can, touch and talk to your baby. Feed and change him. By providing breastmilk you are giving your baby the very best gift you can.

Chapter 51

Breastfeeding and Jaundice

Jaundice is caused by a buildup of bilirubin in the blood. Bilirubin is a yellow pigment which comes from the breakdown of old red blood cells. It is normal for red blood cells to break down, but the bilirubin formed does not usually cause jaundice because the liver metabolizes it and gets rid of it into the gut. The newborn baby, however, often becomes jaundiced during the first few days because the liver enzyme which metabolizes bilirubin is relatively immature. Furthermore, newborn babies have more red blood cells than adults, and thus more are breaking down at any one time. The level of bilirubin in the blood may rise higher than what is usual if the baby:

- is born premature
- is stressed from a difficult birth
- is the infant of a diabetic mother
- has more than the usual number of red blood cells breaking down (as happens in blood incompatibility).

Types of Jaundice

Jaundice Due to Conjugated Bilirubin

The liver changes bilirubin so that it can be eliminated from the body. If, however, the liver is functioning poorly (as occurs during some

Excerpted from Handout 7, "Jaundice" by Jack Newman, M.D., F.R.C.P.C. Revised January 2000. Reprinted with permission.

infections) or the tubes which transport the bilirubin to the gut are blocked, this changed bilirubin may accumulate in the blood and also cause jaundice. When this occurs, the changed bilirubin (called conjugated bilirubin) appears in the urine and turns the urine brown. This brown urine is an important clue that the jaundice is not "ordinary." Jaundice due to conjugated bilirubin is always abnormal, frequently serious, and needs to be investigated thoroughly and immediately. Except in the case of a few extremely rare metabolic diseases, breastfeeding can and should continue.

Physiologic Jaundice

Accumulation of bilirubin before it has been changed by the enzyme of the liver may be normal "physiologic jaundice." Physiologic jaundice begins on the second or third day of life, peaks on the third or fourth day, and then begins to disappear. However, there may be other conditions which cause an exaggeration of this type of jaundice, such as a more rapid than normal breakdown of red blood cells. Because these conditions have no association with breastfeeding, breastfeeding should continue.

Breastmilk Jaundice

There is a condition commonly called breastmilk jaundice. No one knows what the cause of breastmilk jaundice is. In order to make this diagnosis, the baby should be at least a week old, though interestingly, many of the babies with breastmilk jaundice also have had physiologic jaundice, sometimes to levels higher than usual. The baby should be gaining weight well with breastfeeding alone; having lots of bowel movements; passing plentiful, clear urine; and be generally well. In such a setting, the baby has what some call breastmilk jaundice, though, on occasion, infections of the urine or an under functioning of the baby's thyroid gland may cause the same symptoms.

Breastmilk jaundice peaks at ten to twenty-one days, but may last for two to three months. Breastmilk jaundice is normal. Rarely, if ever, does breastfeeding need to be discontinued even for a short time. There is not one bit of evidence that this jaundice causes any problem at all for the baby. Breastfeeding should not be discontinued in order to make a diagnosis. If, however, your doctor feels that discontinuing breastfeeding is appropriate, it would be worth trying a lactation aid with formula rather than taking the baby off the breast altogether, since this may result in difficulties with breastfeeding afterwards. If the baby is truly doing well on breast only, there is no reason to stop breastfeeding or supplement with a lactation aid.

The notion that there is something wrong with the baby being jaundiced comes from the assumption that the formula feeding baby is the standard by which we should determine how the breastfed baby should be. The formula fed baby is rarely jaundiced after the first week of life, and when he is, there is usually something wrong. However, in our experience, most exclusively breastfed babies who are perfectly healthy and gaining weight well are still jaundiced at five to six weeks of life and even later. Do not stop breastfeeding for jaundice.

Not-Enough-Breastmilk Jaundice

Higher than usual levels of bilirubin or longer than usual jaundice may occur because the baby is not getting enough milk. This may be due to the fact that the mother's milk takes a longer than average time to come in, because hospital routines limit breastfeeding, or because the baby is poorly latched on and thus not getting the milk which is available. When the baby is getting little milk, bowel movements tend to be scant and infrequent so that the bilirubin that was in the baby's gut gets reabsorbed into the blood instead of leaving the body with the bowel movements.

Obviously, the best way to avoid "not-enough-breastmilk jaundice" is to get breastfeeding started properly. However, the answer to not-enough-breastmilk jaundice is not to take the baby off the breast or to give bottles. If the baby is nursing well, more frequent feedings may be enough to bring the bilirubin down more quickly, though, in fact, nothing needs be done. If the baby is nursing poorly, helping the baby latch on better may allow him to nurse more effectively and thus receive more milk. Compressing the breast to get more milk into the baby may help. If latching and breast compression alone do not work, a lactation aid would be appropriate to supplement feedings.

Phototherapy (Bilirubin Lights)

Phototherapy increases the fluid requirements of the baby. If the baby is nursing well, more frequent feeding can usually make up this increased requirement. However, if it is felt that the baby needs more fluids, use a lactation aid to supplement; preferably expressed breastmilk, expressed milk with sugar water, or sugar water alone rather than formula should be given.

Chapter 52

Human Milk Banking

A History of Milk Banking

All through history women have provided milk for certain infants whose own mothers were unable to care for them. In the era before the manufacture of commercial infant formula, it was well understood that infants fed on substitutes would likely die. After the industrial revolution, when wet nurses became difficult to find, human milk banking arose. Probably the first such milk bank in the United States was started in 1911 by two Boston physicians who were concerned about the high death rate in an orphan asylum in their community. Over the next decades, advances in the dairy industry helped milk banks develop protocols for sterilizing, pasteurizing, storing, and freezing mothers' milk. In 1943, the American Academy of Pediatrics published its first recommendations for operating human milk banks. A parallel human milk banking tradition arose in Europe, which never embraced infant formula to the extent found in the U.S. In 1959, there were over 100 milk banks in Germany alone.

With aggressive marketing of infant formula, and especially since the onset of the AIDS epidemic, the number of human milk banks has declined. At present there are only a few such institutions operating

This chapter includes text from "A History of Milk Banking," ©1999 Mothers' Milk Bank at Austin, available at http://mmbaustin.org; used with permission. And, "Human Milk Banking," © Lactation Education Resources On-Line, available at http://www.leron-line.com/Milk%20Banking.htm; used with the permission.

in the United States. While the population of infants and children who depend upon donor milk for health and even survival is small, their numbers are greater than the currently existing banks can supply. Additionally, there is increasing evidence that human milk may play an important role in the treatment of some diseases and conditions experienced by older children and adults.

Who Receives Donor Milk?

Recipients are infants who have a medical need for human milk. It is dispensed only on a physician's prescription. Frozen milk can be delivered anywhere in the US via overnight air shipping. Handling fees for pasteurized milk range from $2.00 to $2.75 per ounce which may be covered by third-party payers, and in special circumstances, by WIC or Medicaid.

What Are the Uses of Donor Milk?

Nutritional Uses

- Prematurity
- Failure to thrive
- Malabsorption syndromes
- Short-gut syndrome
- Renal failure
- Feeding intolerance
- Inborn errors of metabolism
- Post-surgical nutrition
- Cardiac problems
- Bronchopulmonary dysplasia
- Pediatric burn cases

Medicinal and Therapeutic Uses of Donor Milk

- Treatment for infectious diseases (intractable diarrhea, gastro-enteritis, infantile botulism, sepsis, pneumonia, hemorrhagic conjunctivitis)

- Post-surgical healing (omphalocele, gastroschisis, intestinal obstruction/bowel fistula, colostomy repair)

- Immunodeficiency diseases (severe allergies, IgA deficiencies)

- Solid organ transplants (including adults)

- Non-infectious intestinal disorders (ulcerative colitis, irritable bowel syndrome)

Preventive Uses of Pasteurized Donor Milk

- Necrotizing enterocolitis
- Crohn's disease
- Colitis
- Allergies to bovine and soy milks/ feeding intolerance
- During immune suppression therapy

Is Donor Milk Safe?

Donors are volunteers who are screened for their health history and have negative blood tests for HIV-1 and 2, Syphilis, Hepatitis B and C, HIV P24, HTLV 1 and 2. Blood testing is done by the milk bank. Human milk is pumped and delivered to the milk bank frozen. There it is thawed, cultured, and pasteurized.

Where Is Donor Milk Available?

Screened, tested, and pasteurized breastmilk is available from the following milk banks who are members of the Human Milk Banking Association of North America, Inc.

Mothers' Milk Bank, Valley Medical Center
P.O. Box 5730
San Jose, CA 95150
Phone: 408-998-4550
Fax: 408-297-9208.

Mother's Milk Bank, P/SL Medical Center
1719 E 19th Ave.
Denver, CO 80218
Phone: 303-869-1888
Fax 303-869-2490

Wilmington Mothers' Milk Bank, Medical Center of Delaware
P.O. Box 1665
Wilmington, DE 19579
Phone: 1-800-642-8101
Fax: 302-733-2602

U Mass Memorial Health Care, Regional Milk Bank
119 Belmont St.
Worcester, MA 01605
Phone: 508-793-6005
Fax: 508-793-5206

Triangle Lactation Center and Milk Bank, WakeMed
3000 New Bern Ave.
Raleigh, NC 27610
Phone: 919-350-8599

Mothers' Milk Bank
900 E 30th St. #101
Austin, TX 78705
Phone: 512-494-0800
Fax: 512-494-0880

Lactation Support Service,
British Columbia Children's Hospital
4480 Oak St., Vancouver, BC V6H 3V4 Canada
Phone: 604-875-2282

Banco de Leche
#2903, C.P. 91020
Xalapa, Veracruz, Mexico
Phone: 52-55-14-45-00

Call the milk bank closest to you for additional details about donating or obtaining donor milk.

References

1. Riordan J and Auerbach K: *Breastfeeding and Human Lactation*. Jones and Bartlett, 1993; p 597.

2. AAP: Recommended standards for the operation of mothers' milk bureaus. *J Pediatrics* 1943; 23:112–28.

3. Springer S: Human milk banking in Germany. *Journal of Human Lactation* 1997; 13(1):6–68.

4. Wiggins P and Arnold L: Clinical case history: Donor milk use for severe gastroespohageal reflux in an adult. *Journal of Human Lactation* 1998; 14(2):157–59.

Chapter 53

Dietary Guidelines for Teenage Mothers

There are Recommended Dietary Allowances, or RDAs, for teenagers and for women nursing a baby. But should there be special nutritional guidelines for teenage mothers who are nursing? Some preliminary research suggests it might be a good idea.

Pediatrician Kathleen Motil, who is with the Agricultural Research Service's Children's Nutrition Research Center in Houston, Texas, compared the milk production of twenty-two mothers—half teens, half adults. The nutrient compositions were similar, but the teens produced 37 to 54 percent less milk than adults. Motil's findings were published last summer in the *Journal of Adolescent Health*.

Motil said the differences between adult and teen milk production remained statistically significant, even after she adjusted the data for differences in feeding time and daily nursing frequency. Why should the milk volume be different? Motil has a theory.

"Our preliminary observations suggest that teenage mothers are facing a dual metabolic challenge," said Motil. "It may be they are still growing, themselves, which may cause an extra nutritional demand."

Motil and her colleagues wanted to find out more about teen nutrition during lactation. They measured body composition, dietary intakes, and milk production. The participants were twenty-four teenage mothers, half of whom breastfed their infants. Eleven additional teens who had never been pregnant served as a control group. Barbara

"Special Dietary Guidelines for Teenage Mothers" by Jill Lee. Reprinted from *Agricultural Research Magazine*, March 1998. Agricultural Research Service, www.ars.usda.gov.

267

Kertz, patient service coordinator at the nutrition research center, organized the study.

Preliminary findings suggest that teenagers who nurse their infants continue to add muscle mass to their bodies, indicating ongoing growth.

"We found that nursing teens consumed more energy (calories), protein, and vitamin B6 than teen mothers who bottle fed or teens who never had children," says Kertz. "They were taking in 23 percent more calories and vitamin B6 and 40 percent more protein." The teens' intake returned to regular levels after weaning. This research team also included nutritionist Corinne Montandon, who helped the girls keep a food journal to track the amounts and kinds of foods they ate. Montandon reviewed the journals for accuracy and sometimes provided a little advice. She cautioned one mother, for example, against trying to crash diet her way back to a pre-pregnancy figure.

Encouraging Breastfeeding

Knowing about teenagers' nutritional demands during breastfeeding fits into a bigger plan of encouraging all mothers to breastfeed—regardless of age. In fact, USDA's Food and Nutrition Service (FNS) has started a nationwide campaign to encourage breastfeeding.

The number of U.S. teenagers becoming pregnant has been declining, but many groups estimate half a million girls under age twenty do give birth annually. For those who choose to raise their infants, breastfeeding can offer advantages such as protection against a broad range of infections and enhanced bonding.

Teenagers are less likely to chose breastfeeding than adults, however. During an FNS focus group on breastfeeding, women of all ages cited embarrassment and lack of family support as barriers to breastfeeding.

But teens face special problems, according to a survey by Alain Joffe, M.D., of the Department of Pediatrics at Johns Hopkins University Hospital. Joffe has studied breastfeeding among 250 inner city teens in Baltimore, Maryland. Susan Radius, a sociologist at nearby Towson University, was a co-author.

The researchers found teenage mothers who returned to high school had a hard time working nursing into their schedule.

Joffe said in his survey the best indicator of whether a teen would breastfeed successfully was having a breastfeeding mentor. That person could be her mother, aunt, or other older friend who had breastfed successfully and could provide advice.

He added that for teens to accept breastfeeding they must know the benefits and feel confident about ways of dealing with obstacles. Some high schools, for example, allow new mothers special time to breastfeed.

Breastfeeding advice and public acceptance seem a long way from research. But these outside factors can have very real effects on the science. In fact, the researchers have to account for the extent of their teenage subjects breastfeeding knowledge. That's why Kertz, a lactational consultant, met with the girls in their study from delivery onward, to provide breastfeeding basics.

Still, the researchers at the Houston center don't know exactly how the teens handled their breastfeeding before their study began. Theresa O. Scholl, who is with the University of Medicine and Dentistry of New Jersey, read Motil's paper on breastmilk production. Scholl's career has focused on the effects of teen pregnancy and lactation on the health of girls and their infants.

"The differences between the growing teens and adult women in this study are huge. It's really impressive," says Scholl. "It might be good to do a follow-up study of the infants from birth to the first 6 months. That way, you could find out if the teen mothers were offering to nurse less often from the start and if that contributed to a reduction in milk flow."

Kertz agrees that the study's findings, like all scientific research, open the door to new questions.

"Breastfeeding is an issue of supply and demand," she says. "The more a mother breastfeeds, the more milk she'll have and the longer she'll be able to nurse. Most of the girls weaned their infants at three to four months. Was this an arbitrary decision to stop nursing, or did the young mothers lack the nutrients to continue?"

There are bigger questions, however—the most basic one being how real is the competition between growing teens and their infants for nutrients? Another is: Do the girls really continue to grow during their childbearing and nursing? Medical textbooks once said no; now the question is being revisited.

Scholl points to her studies of pregnant teens that measured growth of the lower leg only, rather than from head to foot. Lordosis, a natural bending of the spine during pregnancy, can cause errors in a head-to-foot measurement. These studies suggested strongly that growth continues during pregnancy.

Does it follow that continued growth in teens could affect breastmilk volume? Scholl points out that, during pregnancy at least, nature often favors the mother during nutrient stress. Studies on famine and infant birth weight have suggested this natural advantage may have contributed to the survival of the human species.

"Nature wouldn't allow the mother to deplete all her resources," says Scholl. "If it did, she couldn't live to bear more offspring. Moreover, if the mother died, what would happen to her baby?"

More research will need to be done to say with certainty that teen growth causes nutrient competition that results in lower birth weights in newborns and less milk during lactation. But Scholl's work on teen births and Motil's work on teen nursing lend support to the theory that the body puts some of its nutrients on reserve to benefit the teenage mother.

If this proves to be true, physicians will want to be sure that teenage mothers are getting the extra nutrition they and their infants need to ensure breastfeeding success.

Chapter 54

Breastfeeding and the African-American Woman

Why Is Breastfeeding Important for African-American Women?

Nursing mothers and most health care professionals agree that the benefits of breastfeeding are endless. Unfortunately, millions of African-American parents don't take advantage of this form of infant nutrition. The breastfeeding rates of African-American women are markedly lower than White and Hispanic women. In fact, only 19% of African-American women are breastfeeding by the time their babies are six months old. African-American teenagers are even less likely to breastfeed. A hundred years ago, African women in America practiced a tradition of breastfeeding. This tradition should not be forgotten.

Why Are Breastfeeding Rates in the African-American Community So Low?

- Breastfeeding is not seen as "normal" in the African-American community. What could be more normal and natural than breastfeeding?

"An Easy Guide to Breastfeeding for African-American Women," found at www.4woman.gov, was created from a booklet designed and published by the African-American Breastfeeding Alliance, Inc. (AABA), in partnership with the U.S. Office of Health and Human Services Office on Women's Health. Last updated July 2001.

- Breastfeeding is thought to be painful. If done properly, breastfeeding will not cause pain, it will cause joy.

- The African-American community is based on kinship. The decision to breastfeed is directly related to influence from peers (a partner, mother, grandmother, friend, or other relative). It has been found that the African-American woman is very likely to breastfeed if her spouse supports breastfeeding. If her spouse is against breastfeeding, she may be less likely to breastfeed.

- African-Americans don't have access to helpful breastfeeding information. They often go through an entire pregnancy without receiving any information on breastfeeding. Learning the benefits of breastfeeding should be a standard part of prenatal care.

- African-American women are not given a choice about how they want to feed their babies. They are overloaded with coupons, samples, and literature from infant formula companies.

- There are few brochures, posters, or other literature that show pictures of African-American women breastfeeding their babies. There are, however, many brochures and posters that show pictures of White and Hispanic women in breastfeeding situations. This lack of culturally sensitive images has greatly influenced a belief that breastfeeding is no longer a part of the African-American community.

Why Should You Ask Your Doctor about Breastfeeding?

Your doctor should promote breastfeeding as the first choice in infant feeding. Many studies have shown that African-American babies would benefit from breastfeeding because it reduces the community's high incidence of infant mortality and SIDS rates, and is remarkably suited for the health of low-birth weight and premature babies. The benefits of breastfeeding are unparalleled and cannot be duplicated in formula. The American Academy of Pediatrics says,

> "Human milk is uniquely superior for infant feeding. The breast-fed infant is the model against which all alternative-feeding methods must be measured."

It's important for your doctor or health care provider to offer you basic breastfeeding information. Often, African-American women do not receive adequate, or any, information on the importance of breastfeeding.

Feel free to ask your doctor about his or her views on breastfeeding, and on how you can prepare yourself for the experience. You can ask your doctor:

Helpful Questions to Ask at Your Next Doctor's Visit

- How do I prepare myself for breastfeeding?

- Do I need to prepare my breasts before the baby is born?

- Where can I get breastfeeding support?

- How can I become a breastfeeding peer counselor?

- What are the phone numbers of your other breastfeeding patients?

- Any additional questions you may have.

What Is Being Done to Educate African-American Parents about Breastfeeding?

The African-American Breastfeeding Alliance, Inc. (AABA) is the first organization whose sole purpose is to promote breastfeeding to African-American mothers, fathers, and families. AABA's goals are to:

- improve the overall health status of African-American babies,

- increase access to breastfeeding information for African-American parents, and

- create a breastfeeding-friendly culture within the African-American community.

AABA's programs include the African-American Breastfeeding Campaign, Peer Counselor Training, Breastfeeding Hotline, Breast-feeding Drop-In Clinic, Roundtable Discussions, and Comprehensive Research Initiatives services. An emphasis is placed on producing publications and videos that show African-American women breastfeeding their babies. If you would like more information on AABA, call toll-free at 1-877-532-8535.

Chapter 55

Smoking and Breastfeeding

Is It Safe for a Smoker to Breastfeed Her Baby?

Today, most people are aware of the health risks associated with cigarette smoking—both for smokers and for those around them. Pregnancy is often a good incentive for a woman to cut down or quit entirely. If a mother smokes cigarettes, her baby can still enjoy the benefits of breastfeeding. But the more cigarettes a mother smokes, the greater the health risks for both her and her baby—whether he is breastfed or bottle fed.

According to La Leche League International's *Breastfeeding Answer Book*, if the mother smokes fewer than twenty cigarettes a day, the risks to her baby from the nicotine in her milk are small. When a breastfeeding mother smokes more than twenty to thirty cigarettes a day, the risks increase. Heavy smoking can reduce a mother's milk supply and on rare occasions has caused symptoms in the breastfeeding baby such as nausea, vomiting, abdominal cramps, and diarrhea. (Vorherr 1974). By keeping smoking to a minimum, a mother can decrease the risk. When a mother smokes a cigarette, the nicotine levels in her blood and milk first increase and then decrease over time. The half-life of nicotine (the amount of time it takes for half the nicotine to be eliminated from the body) is ninety-five minutes. For this reason, a mother should avoid smoking just before and certainly during a feeding.

"FAQ on Smoking and Breastfeeding," last modified 1999. ©1999 La Leche League International (LLLI), www.lalecheleague.org. Reprinted with permission.

Maternal smoking has been linked to early weaning, lowered milk production, and inhibition of the milk-ejection (let-down) reflex. Smoking also lowers prolactin levels in the blood. One study (Hopkinson et al 1992) clearly suggests that cigarette smoking significantly reduces breast milk production at two weeks postpartum from 514 milliliters per day in non-smokers to 406 milliliters per day in smoking mothers. Mothers who smoke also have slightly higher metabolic rates and may be leaner than non-smoking mothers, therefore, caloric stores for lactation may be low and the mother may need to eat more.

Smoking has been linked to fussiness. In one study, 40% of babies breastfed by smokers were rated as colicky (two to three hours of excessive crying) as compared with 26% of babies breastfed by nonsmokers (Matheson and Rivrud 1989). It's important to note that this link between smoking and colic has also been found with artificially-fed babies with one or more smokers in the home (Lawrence, p.519).

However the baby is fed, parents should avoid exposing him to second-hand smoke by smoking in another room or preferably outside the house. Breathing second-hand or "side-stream" smoke poses health risks. Researchers have documented the health hazards to children when one or both parents smoke. In one study (Colley and Corkhill 1974) researchers monitored the respiratory health of 2,205 babies and found a significant correlation between parents' smoking habits and the incidence of pneumonia, bronchitis, and SIDS during their babies' first year of life. These increased risks are present in both breastfed and bottle-fed infants.

Bottle-fed infants have a much higher incidence of respiratory illnesses than breastfed infants. A bottle-fed baby whose mother or other household members smoke would therefore be at even higher risk of these problems. Dr. Jack Newman states "The risks of not breastfeeding are greater to the baby than the risks of breastfeeding and smoking. The decision is up to the mother and I would encourage her to breastfeed."

What about Using the Nicotine Patch and Other Smoking Cessation Aids?

Due to the highly addictive nature of cigarette smoking, mothers who would like to quit may wonder about the safety of smoking cessation aids which replace nicotine. When used as directed, these products pose no more problems for the breastfeeding infant than maternal smoking does.

According to the 1999 edition of *Medications And Mother's Milk* by Thomas W. Hale, R.Ph., Ph.D., the blood level of nicotine in most smokers (20 cigarettes per day) approaches 44 nanogram per milliliter (ng/mL) whereas levels in patch users average 17 ng/mL, depending on the dose in the patch.

Dr. Hale writes,

> Therefore, nicotine levels in milk can be expected to be less in patch users than those found in smokers, assuming the patch is used correctly and the mother abstains from smoking. Individuals who both smoke and use the patch would have extremely high blood nicotine levels and could endanger the nursing infant. Patches should be removed at bedtime to reduce exposure of the infant and reduce side effects such as nightmares.

> With nicotine gum, maternal serum nicotine levels average 30–60% of those found in cigarette smokers. While patches (transdermal systems) produce a sustained and lower nicotine plasma level, nicotine gum may produce large variations in blood plasma levels when the gum is chewed rapidly, fluctuations similar to smoking itself. Mothers who choose to use nicotine gum and breastfeed should be counseled to refrain from breastfeeding for two to three hours after using the gum product.

Chapter 56

Breastfeeding and Lupus

Twenty years ago, medical textbooks said that women with lupus should not get pregnant because of the risks to both the mother and unborn child. Today, most women with lupus can safely become pregnant. With proper medical care you can decrease the risks associated with pregnancy and deliver a normal, healthy baby.

The most important question that pregnant lupus patients ask is, "Will my baby be okay?" In most cases, the answer is yes. Babies born to women with lupus have no greater chance of birth defects or mental retardation than do babies born to women without lupus. As your pregnancy progresses, the doctor will regularly check the baby's heartbeat and growth with sonograms. About 25% of lupus pregnancies end in unexpected miscarriages or stillbirths. Another 25% may result in premature birth of the infant. Although prematurity presents a danger to the baby, most problems can be successfully treated in a hospital that specializes in caring for premature newborns.

Develop a plan for help at home during the pregnancy and after the baby is born. Motherhood can be overwhelming and tiring, and even more so for a woman with lupus. Although most women with lupus do well, some may become ill and find it difficult to care for their child.

Patient Information Sheet #11, "Pregnancy and Lupus," from *LUPUS: A Patient Care Guide for Nurses and Other Health Professionals*. Published by the National Institute of Arthritis and Musculoskeletal and Skin Diseases (NIAMS) and the National Institutes of Health (NIH), www.nih.gov.

After the Baby Is Born (The Postpartum Period)

Be sure your doctor or nurse reviews with you the physical and emotional changes that occur as your body returns to normal. These changes are the same as those experienced by women who do not have lupus.

Be aware that postpartum complications can arise. In addition to those that can occur to any woman who has been pregnant, you might develop a lupus flare.

Try to breastfeed your baby. It is the ideal, low-cost way to provide nutrition for your baby in the first weeks or months of life. It takes time for mothers and babies to learn how to breastfeed and it may take a few weeks to get adjusted. Because breastfeeding can sometimes be a challenge, ask your doctor or nurse for help so you do not become discouraged. Sometimes, though, breastfeeding may not be possible for the following reasons:

- A premature baby may not be able to suck adequately. Feeding your baby through a tube at first and then by bottle may be necessary. However, you may still be able to pump your breastmilk for your baby. (See Chapter 50, Breastfeeding the Premature Baby.)

- If you are taking corticosteroids, you may not be able to produce enough milk.

- Some medications can pass through your breastmilk to your infant. It will be up to your doctor to decide if breastfeeding is safe if you are taking any of these medications.

- Because breastfed infants tend to eat more frequently than do bottle-fed infants, breastfeeding can be very tiring. You may want to switch to a bottle and formula if breastfeeding becomes too tiring.

Be confident, though, that whichever method you choose to use to feed your baby, it will be the right decision for everyone concerned.

Before you leave the hospital, discuss birth control options with your doctor. Because it would be unwise for you to become pregnant again soon after giving birth, be sure to use an effective birth control method. Remember—you can get pregnant before your period begins again. Also, breastfeeding and withdrawal of the penis before ejaculation are not effective birth control methods.

Caring for Yourself

- Keep all of your appointments with your primary doctor and your obstetrician.

- Get enough rest. Plan for a good night's sleep and rest periods throughout the day.

- Eat a sensible, well-balanced diet. Avoid excessive weight gain. Have your obstetrician refer you to a registered dietitian if necessary.

- Take your medications as prescribed. Your doctor may have you stop some medications and start or continue others.

- Don't smoke, and don't drink alcoholic beverages.

- Be sure your doctor or nurse reviews with you the normal body changes that occur during pregnancy. Some of these changes may be similar to those that occur with a lupus flare. Although it is up to the doctor to determine whether the changes are normal or represent the development of a flare, you must be familiar with them so that you can report them as soon as they occur.

- If you are not sure about a problem or begin to notice a change in the way you feel, talk to your doctor right away.

- Ask your doctor or nurse about participating in childbirth preparation and parenting classes. Although you have lupus, you have the same needs as any other new mother-to-be.

Chapter 57

Breastfeeding and Cancer

While we generally focus on the positive benefits of breastfeeding for the infants, there are additional benefits for the mother as well. Breastfeeding has been found to provide a measure of protection against uterine, cervical, and ovarian cancers as well as breast cancer.

Breast Cancer

A study by Yale University researchers showed that women who breastfed for two years or longer reduced their risk of breast cancer by 50 percent. The researchers studied the medical history of 808 Chinese women in the rural Shandong province from 1997 to 1999. The women were aged 30 to 80 and half had breast cancer and half did not. The study was published in the *American Journal of Epidemiology*. Although the study did not explore the reasons why breastfeeding appears to lower the risk of breast cancer, some researchers say it could be because breastfeeding reduces exposure to estrogen. Yet another theory is that fat-soluble pollutants and carcinogens are not stored as much in lactating breasts as in non-lactating breasts.

In 1999, a group of researchers at the Fred Hutchinson Cancer Research Center in Seattle published the findings of their study of postmenopausal breast cancer risk according to breastfeeding characteristics.

For the study, the researchers contacted 3,633 breast cancer patients aged 50 to 79 from Massachusetts, New Hampshire, and Wisconsin. More than 3,700 women of similar age were randomly selected to serve as the control group. The researchers obtained the women's lactation histories and breast cancer risk factors though telephone interviews.

After adjusting the statistics for age, parity, age at first birth, and other breast cancer risk factors, the researchers found that breast-feeding for at least two weeks was associated with a slightly reduced risk of breast cancer compared to women who have never lactated. Their findings also modestly suggested that women who breastfed longer had a greater reduced risk of breast cancer than those who breastfed for shorter periods of time.

The researchers found no evidence that suggested age at first lactation was associated with breast cancer risk. Also, the use of hormones to suppress lactation was not associated with postmenopausal breast cancer, nor was the inability to breastfed related to risk. The researchers did conclude, however, that lactation may have a slight and perhaps long-lasting protective effect on postmenopausal breast cancer risk. An abstract of this study may be read at the Journal of the American Medical Association's Women's Health Information Center website (www.ama-assn.org/special/womh/womh.htm).

Other Studies

Among both premenopausal and postmenopausal women, risk of breast cancer decrease with increasing duration of lifetime lactation experience although the effect was consistently stronger for premeno-pausal women.

Source: McTieman, A: Evidence of protective effect of lactation on risk of breast cancer in young women. *American Journal of Epidemiology*, 1986.

After controlling for age at first full-term pregnancy and other potentially compounding factors, parity and duration of breastfeeding also had a strong influence on the risk of breast cancer. Compared with parous women who never breastfed, women who had breastfed for twenty-five months or more had a lower relative risk.

Source: Layde, PM: The independent associations of parity age at first full-term pregnancy, and duration of breastfeeding with the risk of breast cancer. *Journal of Clinical Epidemiology*, 1989.

If women who do not breastfeed or who breastfed for less than three months were to do so for four to twelve months, breast cancer among parous premenopausal women could be reduce by 11%; if all women with children lactated for twenty-four months or longer, the incidence might be reduced by nearly 25%.

Source: Newcomb, P et al: Lactation and reduced risk of premenopausal breast cancer. *New England Journal of Medicine* 1994; 330(2):81–87.

Women who were breastfed as infants, even if only for a short time, showed an approximate 25% lower risk of developing premenopausal or postmenopausal breast cancer, compared to women who were bottle-fed as infants.

Source: Freudenheim, J: Exposure to breastmilk in infancy and the risk of breast cancer. *Epidemiology* 1994; 5:324–331.

An increasing duration of lactation was associated with a statistically significant trend toward a reduced risk of breast cancer.

Sources: Newcomb, P.A. et al: Lactation and a reduced risk of premenopausal breast cancer. *New England Journal of Medicine* 1994; 330(2):81–87. P Byers T, et al: Lactation and breast cancer: evidence for a negative association in premenopausal women. *American Journal of Epidemiology* 1985; 121:664–74. Siskind V, et al: Breast cancer and breastfeeding: results from and Australian case-control study. *American Journal of Epidemiology* 1989; 130:229–36.

Other Cancers

Uterine Cancer

A protective effect against uterine cancer was found for women who breastfeed.

Source: Brock, KE: Sexual, reproductive, and contraceptive risk factors for carcinoma-in-situ of the uterine cervix in Sidney. *Medical Journal of Australia* 1989.

Ovarian Cancer

One theory of how breastfeeding may help protect women from ovarian cancer is that breastfeeding reduces the total number of ovulations. The full mechanism by which breastfeeding provides protection is not fully understood, but we can measure the results.

Breastfeeding should be added to the list of factors that decrease ovulatory age and thereby decrease the risk of ovarian cancer.

Source: Schneider, AP: Risk Factors for Ovarian Cancer. *New England Journal of Medicine* 1987.

Endometrial Cancer

Lactation provides a hypoestrogenic effect with less stimulation of the endometrial lining. This event may offer a protective effect from endometrial cancer.

Source: Petterson B, et al: Menstruation span: a time limited risk factor for endometrial carcinoma. *Acta Obstet Gyneocol Scand* 1986; 65:247–55.

Chapter 58

Breastfeeding and the Human Immunodeficiency Virus

The Human Immunodeficiency Virus (HIV) passes via breast-feeding to about one out of seven infants born to HIV-infected women. But in many situations where there is a high prevalence of HIV, the lack of breastfeeding is also associated with a three- to five-fold increase in infant mortality. Infants can die from either the failure to appropriately breastfeed or from the transmission of HIV through breastfeeding.

Furthermore, less than five percent of adults have access to HIV testing. In many countries with high prevalence of HIV, uninfected women may think they have the virus. In the absence of breastfeeding promotion, they may stop breastfeeding even though breastfeeding remains one of the most effective strategies to improve the health and chances of survival of both mother and child.

How Many Infants Are at Risk of HIV?

Analyses of data show that approximately 20 percent of infants born to HIV-infected mothers are infected before or during delivery. If all HIV-infected mothers breastfeed, another 14 percent of their infants will be infected through breastfeeding. This means that about two thirds of children of HIV-infected women will not become infected.

"Breastfeeding and HIV/AIDS: Frequently Asked Questions (FAQ)," a publication of LINKAGES: Breastfeeding, LAM, Complementary Feeding, and Maternal Nutrition Program, www.linkagesproject.org. Updated May 2001, used with permission.

Although the percentage of mothers infected with HIV approaches 40 percent in some African communities, it generally is much lower, rarely above 25 percent (one in four).

The risk of HIV transmission via breastfeeding can be calculated by multiplying the HIV prevalence rate among mothers at the time of delivery (25 percent in the example below) by 14 percent (25 percent at risk x 14 percent infected through breastfeeding = 3.5 percent, or rounded to 4 percent). In other words, even where 25 percent of women are infected with HIV and all of them breastfeed, less than 4 percent of all infants in the community will be infected through breastfeeding.

Should Mothers with HIV Be Advised Not to Breastfeed?

IT DEPENDS . . .

- IF a mother knows she is infected, and
- IF breastmilk substitutes are affordable and can be fed safely with clean water, and
- IF adequate health care is available and affordable,
- THEN the infant's chances of survival are greater if fed artificially.

HOWEVER,

- IF infant mortality is high due to infectious diseases such as diarrhea and pneumonia; or
- IF hygiene, sanitation, and access to clean water are poor; or
- IF the cost of breastmilk substitutes is prohibitively high; or
- IF access to adequate health care is limited;
- THEN breastfeeding may be the safest feeding option even when the mother is HIV-positive.

Even where clean water is accessible, the cost of locally available formula exceeds the average household's income. Families cannot buy sufficient supplies of breastmilk substitutes and tend to:

- over-dilute the breastmilk substitute,
- underfeed their infant, or

- replace the breastmilk substitute with dangerous alternatives.

In the 50 poorest developing countries, infant mortality averages over 100 deaths per thousand live births. Artificial feeding can triple the risk of infant death.

If a Mother with HIV Breastfeeds, How Can She Reduce the Risk of Transmission?

Breastfeeding exclusively for the first six months.

Many experts believe that the safest way to breastfeed in the first six months is to do so exclusively, without adding any other foods or fluids to the infant's diet. These additions are not needed and may cause gut infections that could increase the risk of HIV transmission. In South Africa, mothers who reported exclusively breastfeeding for at least three months were less likely to transmit the virus to their infants than mothers who introduced other foods or fluids before three months. Moreover, their risk of transmitting the virus was no greater than among mothers who never breastfed.

Shortening the total duration of breastfeeding.

There is evidence that the risk of transmission continues as long as the infant is breastfed. The risk of death due to replacement feeding is greatest in the first few months and becomes lower over time. Therefore, in some cases the best strategy may be for a mother to stop breastfeeding early and to introduce breastmilk substitutes as soon as an available replacement method becomes safer. The optimum time and strategy for introducing substitutes, however, is not known and varies with the situation.

Preventing and promptly treating oral lesions and breast problems.

If an infant has oral lesions (commonly caused by thrush) or if a mother has breast problems such as cracked nipples or mastitis, the risk of transmission is higher.

Taking anti-retroviral drugs.

In a recent clinical trial in Uganda, a single dose of nevirapine to a mother during labor and another to her infant after delivery reduced transmission in breastfed infants by 42 percent through six weeks and by 35 percent through twelve months. The simplicity and lower cost of the nevirapine regimen, compared with other regimens that are prohibitively expensive for most poor households, offers hope that it will become an important component of programs to reduce mother-to-child transmission. Studies are being conducted to find out if nevirapine used during the breastfeeding period can further reduce transmission.

What Are the Current International Recommendations on Breastfeeding and HIV?

In May 1997, a policy statement was issued by UNAIDS (the United Nations (UN) system's joint program on HIV/AIDS) whose sponsors include the World Health Organization and UNICEF. The statement, which is supported by technical advisers within USAID and LINKAGES, emphasizes the following:

- supporting breastfeeding in all populations,

- improving access to HIV counseling and testing,

- providing information to empower parents to make fully informed decisions,

- reducing women's vulnerability to HIV infection, and

- preventing commercial pressures to provide artificial feeding.

It also recommends weighing the rates of illness and death from infectious diseases and the availability of safe alternatives to breastfeeding against the risk of HIV transmission when recommending feeding practices. The policy emphasizes the need for parents to make their own infant feeding decisions based on the best available information.

Subsequently, in 1998 the UN agencies published guidelines for policy makers and health care managers to help countries implement this policy. Pilot projects underway in many countries offer voluntary counseling and testing as a part of antenatal services. Pregnant women who test positive for HIV receive counseling on infant feeding options, among other things. To fully understand the positive and negative effects on feeding practices and infant health in the general population, it is important that these efforts are adequately monitored and evaluated. The International Code of Marketing of Breastmilk Substitutes was introduced by the World Health Organization in 1981 to counter the negative effects of the introduction of breastmilk substitutes in developing countries. The Code's provisions are particularly relevant in this era of HIV and should continue to be promoted and observed. The effects of a general reduction in breastfeeding practices would be disastrous for child health and survival.

How Can an Organization Support Breastfeeding While Reducing Mother-to-Child Transmission of HIV?

Promote safer sexual behavior.

The best way of protecting children from HIV is to help women avoid HIV infection. Most infection is through unprotected sexual intercourse. The risk of infection can be decreased by the use of condoms. Methods of protection that women themselves can control are urgently needed. Treating and preventing other sexually transmitted diseases can also help decrease the risk of HIV transmission. Improving the economic and social conditions of women and girls also would reduce their vulnerability to coercive and other unsafe sexual situations.

Provide universal access to voluntary and confidential HIV testing and counseling for both men and women.

At present, testing is not generally available. Many of the strategies proposed for reducing mother-to-child transmission assume that the mother's HIV status is known. Even where testing is available, mothers often do not want to know their status or cannot be assured that test results will be confidential.

Communicate the advantages of knowing one's HIV status.

If a mother knows she is infected, she can try to minimize the risk of transmission to her partners and children and, if she chooses, avoid further pregnancies. As part of her counseling, she should be given information on the risks and benefits of infant feeding options. If she knows she is not infected, she should be counseled to breastfeed, knowing that there is no risk of infecting her child. She should also be motivated to protect herself from further risk of infection. Stimulating demand for testing by emphasizing these advantages along with ensuring the availability of confidential testing is essential.

Provide training to health workers and technical information to opinion makers.

Health care providers and groups with public influence such as the media, policy makers, and health advocates need accurate technical information on this issue to prevent the spread of misinformation and to maintain the strength and credibility of breastfeeding promotion activities.

Provide counseling guidelines to health workers.

UN agencies have developed counseling guidelines for health workers and policy makers that address the risks and benefits of available infant feeding methods and how to make the chosen method of infant feeding as safe as possible. However, until testing programs that help women know their HIV status are available, such guidelines are of limited use.

Continue to promote, protect, and support breastfeeding.

In the absence of breastfeeding promotion, there is a danger that information about HIV transmission during breastfeeding will result in inappropriate discontinuation of breastfeeding among both infected and uninfected mothers. Breastfeeding promotion should include continued efforts to monitor the observance of the provisions of the International Code of Marketing of Breastmilk Substitutes and the use and misuse of information on breastfeeding and HIV.

Support research.

Policies and programs remain hampered by uncertainty. We need to know more about factors that influence transmission rates and about the risks associated with different feeding alternatives in poor environments. Currently, the stage of infection, breastfeeding patterns and duration, related lesions and illness, anti-retroviral therapies, micronutrients, and nutritional status are all being explored as possible influences on transmission. In studies of infant feeding practices, there is a particular need to distinguish different patterns of breastfeeding using standard definitions. We also need to translate this information into knowledge that the mother can use to make the best infant feeding decision for herself, her baby, and her family.

What Advice Can Health Workers Give to Mothers?

Each situation is unique, and health workers must tailor their advice to the individual needs of each mother. Ultimately, the infant feeding choice is the mother's, but this decision should be based on the best information available. The role of the health worker is to provide this information and the support needed to make the mother's choice as safe as possible. Following are counseling guidelines for various situations.

For the woman who is not infected, breastfeeding is clearly the best choice. Breastfeeding remains one of the most effective strategies to improve the health and chances of survival of both the mother and child. It provides a complete and hygienic source of the infant's fluid and nutritional requirements through the first six months of life, as well as growth factors and antibacterial and anti-viral agents that protect the infant from disease for up to two years and more. Breastfeeding also contributes to child spacing and women's long-term health.

HIV and Infant Feeding Counseling Guidelines in Resource-Poor Communities

When the mother's HIV status is unknown, then the health care worker should:

- promote availability and use of confidential testing,
- promote breastfeeding as safer than artificial feeding*, and
- teach the mother how to avoid exposure to HIV.

When the mother is HIV-negative, the health care worker should:

- promote breastfeeding as safest infant feeding method (exclusive breastfeeding for first 6 months, introduction of appropriate complementary foods at about 6 months, and continued breastfeeding to twenty-four months and beyond), and
- teach the mother how to avoid exposure to HIV.

When an HIV-positive mother is considering her feeding options, the health care worker should:

- treat with anti-retroviral drugs, if feasible;
- counsel the mother on the safety, availability, and affordability of feasible infant feeding options;
- help the mother choose and provide safest available infant feeding method; and
- teach mother how to avoid sexual transmission of HIV.

When an HIV-positive mother chooses to breastfeed, the health care worker should:

- promote safer breastfeeding (exclusive breastfeeding up to six months, prevention and treatment of breast problems of mothers and thrush in infants, and shortened duration of breastfeeding when replacements are safe and feasible).

When an HIV-positive mother chooses to feed artificially, the health care worker should:

- help the mother choose the safest alternative infant feeding strategy (methods, timing, etc.), and

- support her in her choice (provide education on hygienic preparation, health care, family planning services, etc.)

*Where testing is not available and where mothers' HIV status is not known, widespread use of artificial feeding would improve child survival only if the prevalence of HIV is high and if the risk of death due to artificial feeding is low, a combination of conditions that does not generally exist.

Does the same advice apply in emergency situations?

The same infant feeding guidelines apply in emergencies. The risk of death due to diarrhea and acute respiratory infections as well as malnutrition is likely to be even greater in emergencies than in normal circumstances.

References

1. Coutsoudis A, Pillay K, Kuhn L, Spooner E, Tsai W-Y, Coovadia HM: Method of feeding and transmission of HIV-1 from mothers to children by 15 months of age: prospective cohort study from Durban, South Africa. *AIDS* 2001; 15:379–387.

2. De Cock KM, Fowler MG, Mercier E, de Vincenzi I, Saba J, Hoff E, Alnwick DJ, Rogers M, Shaffer N: Prevention of mother-to-child HIV transmission in resource-poor countries: Translating research into policy and practice. *JAMA* 2000; 283:1175–1182.

3. Khun L, Stein Z: Infant survival, HIV infection, and feeding alternatives in less-developed countries. *Am J Public Health* 1997; 87:926–931.

4. Nduati R, Ross J: Mother-to-child transmission of HIV through breastfeeding: strategies for prevention. In: Lamptey PR, Gayle H: *HIV/AIDS Prevention and Care in Resource-Constrained Settings: A Handbook for the Management of Programs*. Arlington VA, Family Health International, in press.

5. Nicoll A, Newell M-L, Peckham C, Luo C, Savage F: Infant feeding and HIV-1 infection. *AIDS* 2000; 14(suppl 3):557–574.

6. Preble EA, Piwoz EG: *HIV and Infant Feeding: A Chronology of Research and Policy Advances and their Implications for Programs*. A joint publication of the LINKAGES and Support for Analysis and Research in Africa (SARA) Projects. Washington, DC, Academy for Educational Development,1998.

7. Smith MM, Kuhn L: Exclusive breast-feeding: Does it have the potential to reduce breastfeeding transmission of HIV-1? *Nutr Rev* 2000; 58:333–340.

8. UNAIDS. *HIV and Infant Feeding*. http://www.us.unaids.org/highband/document/epidemio/ infant.html.

8. WHO/UNAIDS/UNICEF. *HIV and Infant Feeding: Guidelines for Decision-makers*. Geneva, World Health Organization, 1998.

9. WHO/UNAIDS/UNICEF. *HIV and Infant Feeding: A Guide for Health Care Managers and Supervisors*. Geneva, World Health Organization, 1998.

Recommendations for Women in the U.S.

The following text is excerpted from, "Public Health Service Task Force Recommendations for the Use of Antiretroviral Drugs in Pregnant Women Infected with HIV-1 for Maternal Health and for Reducing Perinatal HIV-1 Transmission in the United States," *Morbidity and Mortality Weekly (MMWR)*, January 30, 1998. 47(RR-2);1-30. The full text is available on the internet at www.cdc.gov/mmwr/preview/mmwrhtml/00053202.htm.

The U.S. Public Health Service recommends that infected women in the United States refrain from breastfeeding to avoid postnatal transmission of HIV-1 to their infants through breast milk; these recommendations should be followed by women receiving antiretroviral therapy. Passage of antiretroviral drugs into breast milk has been evaluated for only a few antiretroviral drugs. ZDV, 3TC, and nevirapine can be detected in the breast milk of women, and ddI, d4T, and indinavir can be detected in the breast milk of lactating rats. Both the efficacy of antiretroviral therapy for the prevention of postnatal transmission of HIV-1 through breast milk and the toxicity of chronic antiretroviral exposure of the infant via beast milk are unknown.

Applicable Resources

CDC. U.S. Public Health Service Recommendations for human immunodeficiency virus counseling and voluntary testing for pregnant women. *MMWR* 1995;44(RR-7):1-14.

CDC. Recommendations for assisting in the prevention of perinatal transmission of human T-lymphotrophic virus type III/lymphadenopathy-associated virus and acquired immunodeficiency syndrome. *MMWR* 1985;34:721-6.

Chapter 59

When Shouldn't You Breastfeed?

Over the years, many, many, many women have been wrongly told to stop breastfeeding. The decision about continuing breastfeeding when the mother must take a drug, for example, involves more than consideration of whether the medication appears in the mother's milk. It also involves taking into consideration the risks of formula feeding for the baby, which are substantial; the risks of not breastfeeding for the mother, which are substantial; and other issues as well. For example, feeding a breastfeeding baby by bottle for the time the mother is on medication (rarely less than 5 days), will very often result in the baby refusing the breast forever or at least becoming very difficult on the breast. On the other hand, it should be taken into consideration that some babies just will not take bottles, so the advice to stop is not only wrong, but impractical as well. Furthermore, it is easy to advise the mother to pump her milk when she is not feeding the baby, but adequate pumping is often very difficult to do for some mothers, with the result that the mothers may become very painfully engorged, which may further lead to serious complications.

Breastfeeding and Maternal Medication

Most drugs appear in the milk, but only in very tiny amounts. Although a very few drugs may still cause problems for infants even in tiny doses, this is not the case for the vast majority of drugs. Mothers

Excerpted from Handout 9, "You Can Still Breastfeed" by Jack Newman, M.D., F.R.C.P.C. Revised January 1998. Reprinted with permission.

who are told they must stop breastfeeding because of a certain drug should ask to be prescribed an alternative medication which is acceptable for breastfeeding mothers. In this day and age, it is rarely a problem to find such an alternative. If the prescribing physician does not know how to proceed, she should get more information. If the prescribing physician is not flexible, the mother should seek another opinion.

Most drugs may be considered safe for the mother to take and continue breastfeeding if:

1. **They are commonly prescribed for infants.** Examples are amoxycillin, cloxacillin, most antibiotics.

2. **They are considered safe in pregnancy.** Drugs enter directly into the baby's bloodstream when used during pregnancy. The baby generally gets much higher doses at a much more sensitive period during pregnancy than during breastfeeding. However, during pregnancy the mother's liver and kidneys will get rid of the drug for the baby.

3. **They are not absorbed from the stomach or intestines.** These include many drugs which are given by injection. Examples are gentamicin, heparin, lidocaine, or other local anesthetics used by dentists

The following frequently used drugs are also generally safe during breastfeeding: acetaminophen (Tylenol, Tempra), alcohol (in reasonable amounts), aspirin (in usual doses, for short periods), most antiepileptic medications, most antihypertensive medications, tetracycline, codeine, most nonsteroidal anti-inflammatory medications, prednisone, thyroxine, propylthiouracil (PTU), warfarin, tricyclic antidepressant medications, sertraline (Zoloft), paroxetine (Paxil), other antidepressants, metronidazole (Flagyl), Nix, Kwellada.

Medications applied to the skin, inhaled, or applied to the eyes or nose are almost always safe for breastfeeding.

You can still breastfeed after general, regional, or local anesthesia as soon as you are up to it. Medications you might take afterwards for pain are almost always permitted. Immunizations given to the mother do not require her to stop breastfeeding (including with live viruses such as German measles and Hepatitis A and B).

Get reliable information before stopping breastfeeding. Once you have stopped it may be very difficult to restart, especially if the baby is very young.

Breastfeeding and Maternal Illness

Very few maternal illnesses require the mother to stop breast-feeding. This is particularly true of infections. Most infections are caused by viruses. Most infections caused by viruses are most infectious before the mother realizes she is sick. By the time the mother has fever (or cold, runny nose, diarrhea, vomiting, rash, etc.) she has already passed on the infection to the baby. However, breastfeeding protects the baby against infection, and the mother should continue breastfeeding in order to protect the baby. If the baby does get sick, he usually is less sick than if breastfeeding had stopped. But often mothers are pleasantly surprised that their babies do not get sick at all. The baby was protected by his mother's continuing breastfeeding.

The only exception to the above is HIV infection in the mother. Until we have more information, it is considered safer for the baby that the mother who is HIV positive not breastfeed, at least where the risks of bottle feeding are acceptable.

Most other maternal illnesses raise questions because of the drugs the mother might have to take. These should rarely be a problem (see above).

Ordinary X-rays do not require a mother to stop breastfeeding even when used with contrast (e.g. IVP). A CT scan or MRI, even when used with contrast, do not require a mother to stop. A radioactive scan (e.g. lung scan, bone scan) does not require a mother to stop. The only exception is a thyroid scan. However, most of the time the scan does not have to be done. See below.

A not uncommon problem in the early months after delivery is a condition called postpartum thyroiditis, a temporary derangement in the thyroid gland's function. A useful test to help understand the condition is a thyroid scan. However, the test requires that radioactive iodine be given to the mother and this material must not be given to nursing mothers. The radioactive iodine will be found in the milk for weeks, and concentrated in the baby's thyroid. There are ways of dealing with postpartum thyroiditis without doing this test. The drugs a mother might have to take to treat postpartum thyroiditis are compatible with continued breastfeeding (e.g. propranolol, propylthiouracil).

Breast Problems

Mastitis (breast infection) and breast abscess are not reasons to stop breastfeeding. Although surgery on a lactating breast is more difficult, the surgery does not necessarily become easier if the mother stops breastfeeding, as milk continues to be formed for weeks after stopping breastfeeding.

Mammograms are more difficult to read if the mother is breastfeeding, but can still be useful. Once again, how long must a mother wait for her breast no longer to be considered lactating? Evaluation of a lump can be done by other means besides mammography. Discuss options with your doctor. Let him/her know breastfeeding is important to you. A needle biopsy, for example, can be done on a lump which is of concern.

New Pregnancy

There is no reason that you cannot continue breastfeeding if you become pregnant. There is no evidence that this does any harm to you, to the baby in your womb, or to the one who is nursing. If you wish to stop breastfeeding, take your time and wean slowly.

Infant Problems

Breastfeeding rarely needs to be discontinued for infant illness. Through breastfeeding, the mother is able to comfort the sick child, and, at the same time, the child is able to comfort the mother.

1. **Diarrhea and vomiting:** Intestinal infections are rare in exclusively breastfed babies (though loose bowel movements are very common in exclusively breastfed babies). The best treatment for this condition if the baby gets it is to continue breastfeeding. The baby will get better quicker on breastmilk. The baby will do well with only breastmilk in the vast majority of situations, and will not require added fluids except in extraordinary cases.

2. **Respiratory illnesses:** There is a medical myth that milk should not be given to children with respiratory infections. Whether this is true or not for milk, it is definitely not true for breastmilk (and breastfeeding).

3. **Jaundice:** Exclusively breastfed babies are commonly jaundiced, even until the third month, though generally the yellow color of the skin is hardly noticeable. Rather than being a problem, this is normal. (There are causes of jaundice which are not normal, but these do not require stopping breastfeeding). If

breastfeeding is going well, jaundice does not require the baby to stop breastfeeding. If breastfeeding is not going well, fixing the breastfeeding will improve the jaundice. (See Chapter 51, Breastfeeding and Jaundice).

If the question you have is not discussed above, do not assume that you must stop breastfeeding. Do not stop, and get more information.

Part Eight

Additional Help and Information

Chapter 60

Glossary of Terms and Abbreviations

Alternate Breast Massage: *See* Breast Compression.

Alveoli: Tiny glands in the breast which produce milk.[1]

Antibody: A protein substance which combines with an antigen to form the basis of immunity.[1]

Areola: The dark, circular area surrounding the nipple.[1]

Baby Blues: Feelings of melancholy or mild depression common after the birth of a baby. Symptoms of the "baby blues" are less severe and shorter in duration that those of postpartum depression. *See* Postpartum Depression.[3]

Bilirubin: A by-product of the breakdown of the hemoglobin portion of red blood cells. *See* Jaundice.[1]

Bonding: Interaction between parents and infant to form a unique and lasting relationship.[1]

Bottle Feeding: Process by which an infant receives any liquid (including breastmilk) or semi-solid food from a bottle with a nipple or teat.[2]

Terms for this glossary were compiled from the following sources: [1] "Breastfeeding is Best for You and Your Baby Glossary," Public Health—Seattle & King County: Breastfeeding Promotion Project, www.metrokc.gov/ health/breastfeeding; last updated 2001, used with permission. [2] World Health Organization (WHO) Breastfeeding Standard Terminology, definitions last modified 1991, used with permission. And, [3] Definitions written specifically for this volume, ©2002 Omnigraphics, Inc.

Breast Compression (also called Breast Massage, Alternate Breast Massage): Hand massage of the breast used to facilitate letdown and expression of milk.[1]

Breast Infection (also called Mastitis): An inflammation of the breast usually resulting from a plugged duct left untreated or a cracked nipple.[1]

Breast Pump: A device used to express milk from the breasts.[1] Pumps can be electric, battery-operated, or hand powered.[3]

Breastfeeding (also called Nursing): Process by which the infant receives breast milk. The infant may also receive any other food or liquid including non-human milk *See* Exclusive Breastfeeding.[2]

Breastmilk Substitute: Infant formula.[1]

Breast Shell: *See* Breast Shield.

Breast Shield: A hard, round, plastic device that is worn in the bra prenatally to correct inverted nipples. It forms a plastic tent over the areola and encourages flat nipples to protrude during engorgement.[1]

CLE: Certified Lactation Educator

CLC: Certified Lactation Consultant

**CLC: Certified Lactation Counselor

Clutch Hold: *See* Football Hold.

Cradle Hold: Common breastfeeding position in which the baby rests in the mother's arm with his head supported by her elbow and his bottom supported by her hand.[3]

Cross-Cradle Hold: Breastfeeding position for nursing two babies at once. Each baby nurses in the cradle position (*See* Cradle Hold) and the babies' lower bodies cross in the mother's lap.[3]

Colic: Extreme fussiness in the baby which is characterized by a piercing cry, severe abdominal discomfort, and inability to be comforted. This occurs most of the time infant is awake.[1]

Colostrum: Thick yellow or clear fluid secreted from breast during pregnancy and the first few days postpartum before the onset of mature breast milk. It provides nutrients and protection against infectious diseases.[1]

Donor Milk: Breastmilk expressed by a woman unrelated to the baby who will receive it. *See* Human Milk Banking.[3]

Duct System: A system of tubes through which milk flows from the point of production out to the nipple pores.[1]

Engorgement: Swelling and distention of the breasts that may cause discomfort. It is common during the first week of breastfeeding and caused by vascular dilation as well as the arrival of early milk.[1]

Expression: Extracting milk from the breasts, either by hand or by using a breast pump.[1]

Feeding Cues: The ways in which a baby communicates hunger or desire to nurse. Common feeding cues include sucking on fist, increased alertness, and rooting.[3]

Feeding Tube Device (also called Supplemental Nutrition Device, Lactation Aid): A method of supplementing while breastfeeding. A plastic bottle or bag filled with breastmilk or formula hangs from a string around the mother's neck. Thin, soft, plastic tubes lead from the bottle to the mother's nipples. Baby takes tube into his mouth along with the nipple. Commercially available devices are Lact-Aid and Supplemental Nutrition System.[1]

Football Hold (also called Clutch Hold): Common breastfeeding position in which mother cradles the back of the baby's head and neck and the baby's body is supported by the mother's arm. (For example, the baby's head would rest in the mother's right hand, his body would tuck around her right side supported by her right arm. The baby would nurse on the right side.)[3]

Foremilk: Watery, lower-fat, thirst-quenching breastmilk at the beginning of a feed. *See* Hindmilk.[3]

Growth Spurt: A period of sudden growth in the baby when the baby nurses more frequently than usual. Common at three weeks, six to eight weeks, three months, and six months.[1]

Hand Expression: Removal of milk from the breast by manual manipulation.[1]

Hindmilk: Creamy milk that appears after the foremilk. Hindmilk is higher in fat and calories to satisfy a baby's appetite.[3]

Human Milk Banking: Process through which donor milk is collected, screened, and distributed. Recipients include infants, children, and adults with medical conditions that require human milk for nutrition, health, and possibly survival. *See* Donor Milk.[3].

IBCLC: International Board Certified Lactation Consultant

Jaundice: A yellow coloring of the tissues, membranes and secretions due to the presence of bile pigments (bilirubin) in the blood. Physiologic jaundice is a common type of neonatal jaundice resulting from the normal breakdown of red blood cells and the delay in removing their byproducts from the bloodstream. It appears by the third day of life.[1]

Lactation: Breastfeeding; the secretion of breast milk.[1]

Lactation Aid: *See* Feeding Tube Device.

Lactation Professional: Type of health care provider trained in assisting and educating breastfeeding mothers to ensure breastfeeding success and overcome challenges. Lactation professionals can have a variety of credentials and titles including lactation consultant, lactation educator, and breastfeeding counselor.[3]

Latch-on: Process of correctly positioning a baby at the breast to ensure proper sucking.[2]

Leaking: The involuntary release of breast milk.[1]

Letdown Reflex: *See* Milk Ejection Reflex.

Mammary Gland: Breast; gland which secretes milk.[1]

Mastitis: The medical term for a breast infection. *See* Breast Infection.[1]

Milk Ejection Reflex (also called Let Down Reflex): A conditioned reflex ejecting milk from the alveoli through the ducts to the sinuses.[1]

Milk Supply: The quantity of milk a woman produces, usually compared to the baby's requirements for milk.[1]

Nipple: The protruding part of the breast which extends and becomes firmer upon stimulation.[1]

Nipple, Flat: A nipple with a very short shank which does not become erect in response to stimulation.[1]

Nipple, Inverted: A nipple which remains retracted, both when at rest and upon stimulation.[1]

Nipple Confusion: Difficulty in suckling resulting from alternating between breast and bottle feeding which requires two completely different physical actions.[1]

Nipple Pore: Outside opening through which breastmilk flows.[1]

Nipple Shield: An artificial latex or silicone nipple used over the mother's nipple during nursing.[1]

Nipple Transfer Problem: *See* Nipple Confusion.

Nursing Strike: Sudden refusal to breastfeed. Nursing strikes are usually temporary and often related to external factors such as illness, stress, or a change in the baby's environment.[3]

Oxytocin: Hormone that causes milk glands to contract, moving milk into milk ducts.[3]

Plugged Duct: Blockage in a milk duct caused by accumulated milk or cast-off cells.[1]

Postpartum: The 6-week period following childbirth.[1]

Postpartum Depression: Feelings of despondency following the birth of a baby. Postpartum depression can be treated with therapy and/ or medication. *See* Baby Blues.[3]

Predominant Breastfeeding: Requires that the infant receive breast milk (including expressed milk expressed or donor milk) as the predominant source of nourishment. Predominant breastfeeding allows the infant to receive liquids (water, and water-based drinks, fruit, juice, oral rehydration solution), ritual fluids and drops (vitamins, minerals, medicines), however, does not allow the infant to receive anything else (in particular non-human milk, or food-based fluids).[2]

Premature: Infant born before 37 weeks gestation.[1]

Prolactin: Hormone secreted in response to nipple stimulation (baby sucking). Prolactin prepares breasts for milk production and encourages continuous milk production. [3]

Relactation: Process by which a woman who has given birth but did not initially breastfeed is stimulated to lactate. Also applies to reinstituting lactation after it had been discontinued.[1]

Rooting Reflex: The natural instinct of the newborn to turn his head toward the stimulation when touched on the cheek.[1]

Side-Lying Position: Breastfeeding position (similar to the cradle hold) in which the mother lays on her side facing the baby, supporting his body as needed with her arm. This position is especially helpful after birth (especially a surgical birth) or when nursing at night. *See* Cradle Hold.[3]

Sinus: Enlarged portion of the duct where breastmilk pools during letdown. It lies directly behind the areola and connects to nipple pore.[1]

Spitting Up: Baby expelling small amount of milk from the mouth during or after feedings; common in most babies.[1]

Suck: To draw fluid into the mouth by forming a partial vacuum with the lip and tongue. Sucking can be non-nutritive (sucking without swallowing) or nutritive, when milk is swallowed with each suckle.[1]

Suckling: The entire process of an infant breastfeeding; including sucking, compression of areola with jaws, seal with lips, and tongue massaging milk out of the sinuses.[1]

Supplementation: Anything given in addition to breastmilk.[1]

Supplementary Bottle: A routine bottle given in addition to breastfeeding.[1]

Supply and Demand: The process by which the baby's suckling or other stimulation (i.e., hand expression or pumping) controls the amount of milk produced.[1]

Tandem Nursing: Breastfeeding two or more siblings at the same time.[3]

Thrush: A fungal infection of the mouth characterized by white patches and ulcers; candida infection may also occur on mother's nipples.[1]

Vomiting: Expelling the contents of the stomach with force.[1]

Weaning: Discontinuation of breastfeeding by substituting other nourishment.[1]

Chapter 61

Medications and Breastfeeding

The following medicines, selected from those included in *Advice for the Patient: Drug Information in Lay Language* (MICROMEDEX Thomson Healthcare, ©2001), have specific precautions in regard to use while breastfeeding.

The use of any medicine while breastfeeding must be carefully considered. The physician and the patient must balance the expected benefits against the possible risks.

Absence of a drug from this list is not meant to imply that it is safe for use while breastfeeding. For many drugs, it is not known whether a problem exists; experimentation on women who are breastfeeding is generally not done. Knowledge is usually gained only from the accumulated experience over many years in giving a drug to breastfeeding women who needed its benefits. Also, well-planned studies in breastfeeding animals may reveal problems, although the relation of such findings to humans may not be known. Problems suggested by animal studies are often included in the warnings [given for specific drugs in the book *Advice for the Patient: Drug Information in Lay Language, Volume II*].

Readers are reminded that the information in this text is selected and not considered to be complete.

The following information is reprinted with permission:

From Appendix VI "Breast-Feeding Precaution List," *Advice for the Patient: Drug Information in Lay Language Volume II*, USP DI® 21st Edition, © 2001 MICROMEDEX Thomson Healthcare, content prepared by United States Pharmacopeial Convention; reprinted with permission.

A

Acarbose (Systemic)
Acebutolol (Systemic)
Acenocoumarol (Systemic)
Acitretin (Systemic)
Acrivastine (Systemic)
Acrivastine and Pseudoephedrine
    (Systemic)
Alatrofloxacin (Systemic)
Albendazole (Systemic)
Albumin Microspheres Sonicated
    (Systemic)
Albuterol (Inhalation)
Alclometasone (Topical)
Aldesleukin (Systemic)
Alendronate (Systemic)
Alitretinoin (Topical)
Alprazolam (Systemic)
Altretamine (Systemic)
Amantadine (Systemic)
Amcinonide (Topical)
Amiloride and Hydrochlorothiazide
    (Systemic)
Aminophylline (Systemic)
Amiodarone (Systemic)
Amlexanox (Mucosal-Local)
Amlodipine and Benazepril (Sys-
    temic)
Ammonia N 13 (Diagnostic)
Amobarbital (Systemic)
Amoxicillin (Systemic)
Amoxicillin and Clavulanate (Systemic)
Amphetamine (Systemic)
Amphotericin B Cholesteryl Complex
    (Systemic)
Amphotericin B Lipid Complex (Sys-
    temic)
Amphotericin B Liposomal Complex
    (Systemic)
Ampicillin (Systemic)
Ampicillin and Sulbactam (Systemic)
Amprenavir (Systemic)
Amyl Nitrate (Systemic)
Anagrelide (Systemic)
Anastrazole (Systemic)
Anistropine (Systemic)
Apraclonidine (Ophthalmic)

Aprobarbital (Systemic)
Asparaginase (Systemic)
Aspirin (Systemic)
Aspirin, Buffered (Systemic)
Aspirin and Caffeine
Aspirin and Caffeine, Buffered (Sys-
    temic)
Aspirin, Caffeine, and
    Dihydrocodeine (Systemic)
Aspirin and Codeine (Systemic)
Aspirin, Codeine, and Caffeine (Sys-
    temic)
Aspirin, Codeine, and Caffeine, Buff-
    ered (Systemic)
Astemizole (Systemic)
Atenolol (Systemic)
Atenolol and Chlorthalidone (Sys-
    temic)
Atorvastatin (Systemic)
Atropine (Ophthalmic)
Atropine (Systemic)
Atropine, Hyoscyamine, Scopolamine,
    and Phenobarbital (Systemic)
Atropine and Phenobarbital (Sys-
    temic)
Auranofin (Systemic)
Aurothioglucose (Systemic)
Azatadine (Systemic)
Azatadine and Pseudoephedrine (Sys-
    temic)
Azathioprine (Systemic)

B

Bacampicillin (Systemic)
Baclofen (Intrathecal-Systemic)
Baclofen (Systemic)
Basilixumab (Systemic)
Beclomethasone (Topical)
Belladonna (Systemic)
Belladonna and Butabarbital (Sys-
    temic)
Belladonna and Phenobarbital (Sys-
    temic)
Bendroflumethiazide (Systemic)
Benzphetamine (Systemic)
Benztropine (Systemic)
Benzyl Benzoate (Topical)

Betamethasone (Otic)
Betamethasone (Rectal)
Betamethasone (Systemic)
Betamethasone (Topical)
Betaxolol (Systemic)
Bexarotene (Systemic)
Biperiden (Systemic)
Bismuth Subsalicylate (Oral)
Bismuth Subsalicylate, Metronidazole and Tetracycline-for H. pylori (Systemic)
Bisoprolol (Systemic)
Bisoprolol and Hydrochlorothiazide (Systemic)
Bleomycin (Systemic)
Brinzolamide (Ophthalmic)
Bromazepam (Systemic)
Bromocriptine (Systemic)
Bromodiphenhydramine (Systemic)
Bromodiphenhydramine and Codeine (Systemic)
Bromodiphenhydramine, Diphenhydramine, Codeine, Ammonium Chloride, and Potassium Guaiacolsulfonate (Systemic)
Brompheniramine (Systemic)
Brompheniramine and Phenylephrine (Systemic)
Brompheniramine, Phenylephrine, and Phenylpropanolamine (Systemic)
Brompheniramine, Phenylephrine, Phenylpropanolamine, and Codeine (Systemic)
Brompheniramine, Phenylephrine, Phenylpropanolamine, Codeine, and Guaifenesin (Systemic)
Brompheniramine, Phenylephrine, Phenylpropanolamine, and Dextromethorphan (Systemic)
Brompheniramine, Phenylephrine, Phenylpropanolamine, and Guaifenesin (Systemic)
Brompheniramine, Phenylephrine, Phenylpropanolamine, Hydrocodone, and Guaifenesin (Systemic)
Brompheniramine and Phenylpropanolamine (Systemic)

Brompheniramine, Phenylpropanolamine, and Acetaminophen (Systemic)
Brompheniramine, Phenylpropanolamine, and Codeine (Systemic)
Brompheniramine, Phenylpropanolamine, and Dextromethorphan (Systemic)
Brompheniramine and Pseudoephedrine (Systemic)
Brompheniramine, Pseudoephedrine, and Acetaminophen (Systemic)
Brompheniramine, Pseudoephedrine, and Dextromethorphan (Systemic)
Buclizine (Systemic)
Budesonide (Rectal)
Budesonide (Systemic)
Buprenorphine (Systemic)
Bupropion (Systemic)
Busulfan (Systemic)
Butabarbital (Systemic)
Butalbital and Acetaminophen (Systemic)
Butalbital, Acetaminophen, and Caffeine (Systemic)
Butalbital, Acetaminophen, Caffeine, and Codeine (Systemic)
Butalbital and Aspirin (Systemic)
Butalbital, Aspirin, and Caffeine (Systemic)
Butalbital, Aspirin, Caffeine, and Codeine (Systemic)

C

Cabergoline (Systemic)
Caffeine (Systemic)
Caffeine and Sodium Benzoate (Systemic)
Calcitonin (Nasal-Systemic)
Calcitonin-Human (Systemic)
Calcitonin-Salmon (Systemic)
Candesartan (Systemic)
Capecitabine (Systemic)
Carbamazepine (Systemic)
Carbenicillin (Systemic)
Carbidopa and Levodopa (Systemic)

Carbinoxamine (Systemic)

Carbinoxamine and Pseudoephedrine (Systemic)

Carbinoxamine, Pseudoephedrine, and Dextromethorphan (Systemic)

Carboplatin (Systemic)

Carisoprodol (Systemic)

Carmustine (Implantation-Local)

Carmustine (Systemic)

Carteolol (Systemic)

Carvedilol (Systemic)

Cascara Sagrada (Oral)

Cascara Sagrada and Aloe (Oral)

Cascara Sagrada and Phenolphthalein (Oral)

Celecoxib (Systemic)

Cerivastatin (Systemic)

Cetirizine (Systemic)

Chloral Hydrate (Systemic)

Chlorambucil (Systemic)

Chloramphenicol (Otic)

Chloramphenicol (Systemic)

Chlordiazepoxide (Systemic)

Chlordiazepoxide and Amitriptyline (Systemic)

Chlordiazepoxide and Clidinium (Systemic)

Chloroquine (Systemic)

Chlorothiazide (Systemic)

Chlorpheniramine and Codeine (Systemic)

Chlorpheniramine and Dextromethorphan (Systemic)

Chlorpheniramine, Ephedrine, and Guaifenesin (Systemic)

Chlorpheniramine, Ephedrine, Phenylephrine, Dextromethorphan, Ammonium Chloride, and Ipecac (Systemic)

Chlorpheniramine and Hydrocodone (Systemic)

Chlorpheniramine, Phenindamine, Phenylephrine, Dextromethorphan, Acetaminophen, Salicylamide, Caffeine, and Ascorbic Acid (Systemic)

Chlorpheniramine, Phenindamine, and Phenylpropanolamine (Systemic)

Chlorpheniramine, Pheniramine, Pyrilamine, Phenylephrine, Hydrocodone, Salicylamide, Caffeine, and Ascorbic Acid (Systemic)

Chlorpheniramine and Phenylephrine (Systemic)

Chlorpheniramine, Phenylephrine, and Acetaminophen (Systemic)

Chlorpheniramine, Phenylephrine, Codeine, and Ammonium Chloride (Systemic)

Chlorpheniramine, Phenylephrine, Codeine, and Potassium Iodide (Systemic)

Chlorpheniramine, Phenylephrine, and Salicylamide (Systemic)

Chlorpheniramine, Phenylephrine, Dextromethorphan, and Guaifenesin (Systemic)

Chlorpheniramine, Phenylephrine, Dextromethorphan, Guaifenesin, and Ammonium Chloride (Systemic)

Chlorpheniramine, Phenylephrine, and Guaifenesin (Systemic)

Chlorpheniramine, Phenylephrine, and Hydrocodone (Systemic)

Chlorpheniramine, Phenylephrine, Hydrocodone, Acetaminophen, and Caffeine (Systemic)

Chlorpheniramine, Phenylephrine, and Methscopolamine (Systemic)

Chlorpheniramine, Phenylephrine, and Phenylpropanolamine (Systemic)

Chlorpheniramine, Phenylephrine, Phenylpropanolamine, Atropine, Hyoscyamine, and Scopolamine (Systemic)

Chlorpheniramine, Phenylephrine, Phenylpropanolamine, Carbetapentane, and Potassium Guaiacolsulfonate (Systemic)

Chlorpheniramine, Phenylephrine, Phenylpropanolamine, and Codeine (Systemic)

Chlorpheniramine, Phenylephrine, Phenylpropanolamine, Dextromethorphan, Potassium Guaiacolsulfonate, and Ipecac (Systemic)

Chlorpheniramine, Phenylephrine, Phenylpropanolamine, and Dihydrocodeine (Systemic)

Chlorpheniramine and Phenylpropanolamine (Systemic)

Chlorpheniramine, Phenylpropanolamine, and Acetaminophen (Systemic)

Chlorpheniramine, Phenylpropanolamine, Acetaminophen, and Caffeine (Systemic)

Chlorpheniramine, Phenylpropanolamine, and Aspirin (Systemic)

Chlorpheniramine, Phenylpropanolamine, and Caramiphen (Systemic)

Chlorpheniramine, Phenylpropanolamine, and Dextromethorphan (Systemic)

Chlorpheniramine, Phenylpropanolamine, Dextromethorphan, and Acetaminophen (Systemic)

Chlorpheniramine, Phenylpropanolamine, Dextromethorphan, and Aspirin (Systemic)

Chlorpheniramine, Phenylpropanolamine, and Guaifenesin (Systemic)

Chlorpheniramine, Phenylpropanolamine, Guaifenesin, and Acetaminophen (Systemic)

Chlorpheniramine, Phenylpropanolamine, Guaifenesin, Sodium Citrate, and Citric Acid (Systemic)

Chlorpheniramine, Phenylpropanolamine, and Methscopolamine (Systemic)

Chlorpheniramine, Phenylpropanolamine, Ephedrine, Codeine, and Guaiacol Carbonate (Systemic)

Chlorpheniramine, Phenylpropanolamine, and Phenylephrine (Systemic)

Chlorpheniramine, Phenylpropanolamine, Phenylephrine, and Phenylpropanolamine (Systemic)

Chlorpheniramine, Phenylpropanolamine, Phenylpropanolamine, and Acetaminophen (Systemic)

Chlorpheniramine and Pseudoephedrine (Systemic)

Chlorpheniramine, Pseudoephedrine, and Acetaminophen (Systemic)

Chlorpheniramine, Pseudoephedrine, and Codeine (Systemic)

Chlorpheniramine, Pseudoephedrine, Codeine, and Acetaminophen (Systemic)

Chlorpheniramine, Pseudoephedrine, and Dextromethorphan (Systemic)

Chlorpheniramine, Pseudoephedrine, Dextromethorphan, and Acetaminophen (Systemic)

Chlorpheniramine, Pseudoephedrine, Dextromethorphan, and Guaifenesin (Systemic)

Chlorpheniramine, Pseudoephedrine, and Guaifenesin (Systemic)

Chlorpheniramine, Pseudoephedrine, and Hydrocodone (Systemic)

Chlorpheniramine, Pseudoephedrine, and Methscopolamine (Systemic)

Chlorpheniramine, Pyrilamine, and Phenylephrine (Systemic)

Chlorpheniramine, Pyrilamine, Phenylephrine, and Acetaminophen (Systemic)

Chlorpheniramine, Pyrilamine, Phenylephrine, and Phenylpropanolamine (Systemic)

Chlorpheniramine, Pyrilamine, Phenylephrine, Phenylpropanolamine, and Acetaminophen (Systemic)

Chlorpromazine (Systemic)

Chlorpropamide (Systemic)

Chlorprothixene (Systemic)

Chlorthalidone (Systemic)

Cholestyramine (Oral)

Choline Salicylate (Systemic)

Choline and Magnesium Salicylates (Systemic)

Chromic Phosphate P 32 (Therapeutic)]

Cilostazol (Systemic)

Cimetidine (Systemic)

Cinoxacin (Systemic)
Ciprofloxacin (Systemic)
Cisapride (Systemic)
Cisplatin (Systemic)
Citalopram (Systemic)
Cladribine (Systemic)
Clemastine (Systemic)
Clemastine and Phenylpropanola-
    mine (Systemic)
Clidinium (Systemic)
Clobazam (Systemic)
Clobetasol (Topical)
Clobetasone (Topical)
Clocortolone (Topical)
Clofazimine (Systemic)
Clofibrate (Systemic)
Clomiphene (Systemic)
Clonazepam (Systemic)
Clonidine (Parenteral-Local)
Clonidine and Chlorthalidone (Sys-
    temic)
Clorazepate (Systemic)
Clotrimazole and Betamethasone
    (Topical)
Cloxacillin (Systemic)
Clozapine (Systemic)
Cocaine (Mucosal-Local)
Codeine, Ammonium Chloride, and
    Guaifenesin (Systemic)
Codeine and Calcium Iodide (Systemic)
Codeine and Guaifenesin (Systemic)
Codeine and Iodinated Glycerol (Sys-
    temic)
Conjugated Estrogens (Systemic)
Conjugated Estrogens and
    Medroxyprogesterone (Systemic)
Cortisone (Systemic)
Cyanocobalamin Co 57 (Diagnostic)
Cyclizine (Systemic)
Cyclophosphamide (Systemic)
Cyclosporine (Systemic)
Cyproheptadine (Systemic)
Cytarabine (Systemic)
Cytarabine, Liposomal (Intrathecal)

D

Dacarbazine (Systemic)

Daclizumab (Systemic)
Dactinomycin (Systemic)
Danazol (Systemic)
Danthron and Docusate (Oral)
Dantrolene (Systemic)
Dapsone (Systemic)
Daunorubicin (Systemic)
Daunorubicin, Liposomal (Systemic)
Delavirdine (Systemic)
Demecarium (Ophthalmic)
Demeclocycline (Systemic)
Denileukin (Systemic)
Deserpidine (Systemic)
Deserpidine and Methyclothiazide
    (Systemic)
Desflurane (Inhalation-Systemic)
Desmopressin (Systemic)
Desogestrel and Ethinyl Estradiol
    (Systemic)
Desonide (Topical)
Desoximetasone (Topical)
Dexamethasone (Nasal)
Dexamethasone (Otic)
Dexamethasone (Systemic)
Dexamethasone (Topical)
Dexbrompheniramine and Pseu-
    doephedrine (Systemic)
Dexbrompheniramine, Pseudoephe-
    drine, and Acetaminophen (Sys-
    temic)
Dexchlorpheniramine (Systemic)
Dexchlorpheniramine, Pseudoephe-
    drine, and Guaifenesin (Sys-
    temic)
Dextromethorphan and Acetami-
    nophen (Systemic)
Dextromethorphan and Guaifenesin
    (Systemic)
Dextromethorphan and Iodinated
    Glycerol (Systemic)
Diatrizoate and Iodipamide (Diagnos-
    tic, Local)
Diatrizoate Meglumine (Local)
Diatrizoate Sodium (Local)
Diatrizoates (Diagnostic)
Diazepam (Systemic)
Dichlorphenamide (Systemic)
Diclofenac and Misoprostol (Systemic)

Dicloxacillin (Systemic)
Dicyclomine (Systemic)
Dienestrol (Vaginal)
Diethylpropion (Systemic)
Diethylstilbestrol (Systemic)
Diethylstilbestrol and Methyltest-
osterone (Systemic)
Difenoxin and Atropine (Systemic)
Diflorasone (Topical)
Diflucortolone (Topical)
Digitoxin (Systemic)
Digoxin (Systemic)
Dihydroergotamine (Nasal-Systemic)
Dihydroergotamine (Systemic)
Dimenhydrinate (Systemic)
Diphenhydramine (Systemic)
Diphenhydramine, Codeine, and Am-
monium Chloride (Systemic)
Diphenhydramine,
Dextromethorphan, and Ammo-
nium Chloride (Systemic)
Diphenhydramine, Phenylpropanola-
mine, and Aspirin (Systemic)
Diphenhydramine and Pseudoephe-
drine (Systemic)
Diphenhydramine, Pseudoephedrine,
and Acetaminophen (Systemic)
Diphenoxylate and Atropine (Sys-
temic)
Diphenylpyraline (Systemic)
Diphenylpyraline, Phenylephrine,
and Dextromethorphan (Sys-
temic)
Diphenylpyraline, Phenylpropanola-
mine, Acetaminophen, and Caf-
feine (Systemic)
Diphtheria and Tetanus Toxoide (Sys-
temic)
Dipyridamole-Therapeutic (Systemic)
Disopyramide (Systemic)
Divalproex (Systemic)
Docetaxel (Systemic)
Donepezil (Systemic)
Dorzolamide (Ophthalmic)
Dorzolamide and Timolol (Oph-
thalmic)
Doxazosin (Systemic)
Doxepin (Systemic)

Doxepin (Topical)
Doxorubicin (Systemic)
Doxorubicin, Liposomal (Systemic)
Doxycycline (Dental)
Doxycycline (Systemic)
Doxycycline-for dental use (Systemic)
Doxylamine (Systemic)
Doxylamine, Codeine, and Acetami-
nophen (Systemic)
Doxylamine, Etafedrine, and
Hydrocone (Systemic)
Doxylamine, Phenylpropanolamine,
Dextromethorphan, and Aspirin
(Systemic)
Doxylamine, Pseudoephedrine,
Dextromethorphan, and Acetami-
nophen (Systemic)
Dronabinol (Systemic)
Droperidol (Systemic)

E

Echothiophate (Ophthalmic)
Econazole (Topical)
Efavirenz (Systemic)
Enoxacin (Systemic)
Ephedrine (Oral/Injection)
Ephedrine, Carbetapentane, and
Guaifenesin (Systemic)
Ephedrine and Guaifenesin (Systemic)
Ephedrine and Potassium Iodide
(Systemic)
Epinephrine (Inhalation)
Epirubicin (Systemic)
Epoprostenol (Systemic)
Eprosartan (Systemic)
Ergonovine (Systemic)
Ergotamine (Systemic)
Ergotamine, Belladonna Alkaloids,
and Phenobarbital (Systemic)
Ergotamine and Caffeine (Systemic)
Ergotamine, Caffeine, and Bella-
donna Alkaloids (Systemic)
Ergotamine, Caffeine, Belladonna Al-
kaloids, and Pentobarbital (Sys-
temic)
Ergotamine, Caffeine, and Cyclizine
(Systemic)

317

Ergotamine, Caffeine, and Dimenhy-
drinate (Systemic)
Ergotamine, Caffeine, and Diphenhy-
dramine (Systemic)
Eythromycin and Sulfisoxazole (Sys-
temic)
Estazolam (Systemic)
Estradiol (Systemic)
Estradiol (Vaginal)
Estrogens, Conjugated (Systemic)
Estrogens, Conjugated (Vaginal)
Estrogens, Conjugated, and Methylt-
estosterone (Systemic)
Estrogens, Esterified (Systemic)
Estrogens, Esterified, and Methyltes-
tosterone (Systemic)
Estrone (Systemic)
Estrone (Vaginal)
Estropipate (Systemic)
Estropipate (Vaginal)
Etanercept (Systemic)
Ethchlorvynol (Systemic)
Ethinyl Estradiol (Systemic)
Ethopropazine (Systemic)
Ethotoin (Systemic)
Ethynodiol Diacetate and Ethinyl Es-
tradiol (Systemic)
Etoposide (Systemic)
Exemestane (Systemic)

F

Famciclovir (Systemic)
Famotidine (Systemic)
Fenofibrate (Systemic)
Fentanyl (Transdermal-Systemic)
Fentanyl Citrate (Systemic)
Ferrous Citrate Fe 59 (Diagnostic)
Ferumoxides (Diagnostic)
Fexofenadine and Pseudoephedrine
(Systemic)
Finasteride (Systemic)
Flecainide (Systemic)
Floxuridine (Systemic)
Flucloxacillin (Systemic)
Flucytosine (Systemic)
Fludarabine (Systemic)
Fludeoxyglucose F 18 (Diagnostic)

Fludrocortisone (Systemic)
Flumethasone (Topical)
Fluocinolone (Topical)
Fluocinonide (Topical)
Fluorouracil (Systemic)
Fluorouracil (Topical)
Fluoxetine (Systemic)
Fluoxymesterone (Systemic)
Fluoxymesterone and Ethinyl Estra-
diol (Systemic)
Flupenthixol (Systemic)
Fluphenazine (Systemic)
Flurandrenolide (Topical)
Flurazepam (Systemic)
Fluticasone (Nasal)
Fluticasone (Topical)
Fluvastatin (Systemic)
Foscarnet (Systemic)
Fosphenytoin (Systemic)
Furazolidone (Oral)

G

Gadopentetate (Diagnostic)
Gadoversetamide (Systemic)
Gallium Citrate Ga 67 (Diagnostic)
Gallium Nitrate (Systemic)
Ganciclovir (Implantation-Oph-
thalmic)
Ganciclovir (Systemic)
Gemcitabine (Systemic)
Gemfibrozil (Systemic)
Glimepiride (Systemic)
Glutethimide (Systemic)
Glycopyrrolate (Systemic)
Gold Sodium Thiomalate (Systemic)
Goserelin (Systemic)
Guanethidine (Systemic)

H

Halazepam (Systemic)
Halcinonide (Topical)
Halobetasol (Topical)
Halofantrine (Systemic)
Haloperidol (Systemic)
Heparin (Systemic)
Histrelin (Systemic)

Homatropine (Systemic)
Hydralazine (Systemic)
Hydralazine and Hydrochlorothiazide (Systemic)
Hydrochlorothiazide (Systemic)
Hydrocodone and Aspirin (Systemic)
Hydrocodone and Guaifenesin (Systemic)
Hydrocodone and Homatropine (Systemic)
Hydrocodone and Potassium Guaiacolsulfonate (Systemic)
Hydrocortisone (Dental)
Hydrocortisone (Rectal)
Hydrocortisone (Systemic)
Hydrocortisone (Topical)
Hydrocortisone Acetate (Topical)
Hydrocortisone Butyrate (Topical)
Hydrocortisone Valerate (Topical)
Hydroflumethiazide (Systemic)
Hydromorphone and Guaifenesin (Systemic)
Hydroxychloroquine (Systemic)
Hydroxyprogesterone (Systemic)
Hydroxyurea (Systemic)
Hydroxyzine (Systemic)
Hyoscyamine (Systemic)
Hyoscyamine and Phenobarbital (Systemic)

I

Idarubicin (Systemic)
Ifosfamide (Systemic)
Indinavir (Systemic)
Indium in 111 Oxyquinoline (Diagnostic)
Indium in 111 Pentetate (Diagnostic)
Indium in 111 Pentetreotide (Diagnostic)
Indium in 111 Satumomab Pendetide (Diagnostic)
Indomethacin (Systemic)
Infliximab (Systemic)
Insulin (Systemic)
Insulin Human (Systemic)
Insulin Human, Buffered (Systemic)
Insulin, Isophane (Systemic)

Insulin, Isophane, Human (Systemic)
Insulin, Isophane, Human, and Insulin Human (Systemic)
Insulin Lispro (Systemic)
Insulin Zinc (Systemic)
Insulin Zinc, Extended (Systemic)
Insulin Zinc, Extended, Human (Systemic)
Insulin Zinc, Human (Systemic)
Insulin Zinc, Prompt (Systemic)
Interferon Alfa-2a, Recombinant (Systemic)
Interferon Alfa-2v, Recombinant (Systemic)
Interferon Alfacon-1 (Systemic)
Interferon Alfa-n1 (Ins) (Systemic)
Interferon Alfa-n3 (Systemic)
Interferon Beta-1a (Systemic)
Interferon Beta-1b (Systemic)
Interferon, Gamma (Systemic)
Iobenguane, Radioiodinated (Diagnostic)
Iobenguane, Radioiodinated (Therapeutic)
Iocetamic Acid (Diagnostic)
Iodine (Topical)
Iodine, Strong (Systemic)
Iodipamide (Diagnostic)
Iodohippurate Sodium I 123 (Diagnostic)
Iodohippurate Sodium I 131 (Diagnostic)
Iofetamine I 123 (Diagnostic)
Iohexol (Diagnostic)
Iohexol (Diagnostic, Local)
Iopamidol (Diagnostic)
Iopanoic Acid (Diagnostic)
Iothalamate (Diagnostic)
Iothalamate (Diagnostic, Local)
Iothalamate Sodium I 125 (Diagnostic)
Ioversol (Diagnostic)
Ioxaglate (Diagnostic)
Ioxaglate (Diagnostic, Local)
Ipodate (Diagnostic)
Irbesartan (Systemic)
Irinotecan (Systemic)
Isoflurophate (Ophthalmic)

Isoniazid (Systemic)
Isotretinoin (Systemic)

K

Kaolin, Pectin and Paregoric (Systemic)
Ketazolam (Systemic)
Ketorolac (Systemic)
Krypton Kr 81m (Diagnostic)

L

Labetalol (Systemic)
Lamivudine and Zidovudine (Systemic)
Lamotrigine (Systemic)
Lansoprazole (Systemic)
Leflunomide (Systemic)
Letrozole (Systemic)
Leuprolide (Systemic)
Levalbuterol (Inhalation-Local)
Levodopa (Systemic)
Levofloxacin (Systemic)
Levonorgestrel and Ethinyl Estradiol (Systemic)
Lindane (Topical)
Lithium (Systemic)
Lomefloxacin (Systemic)
Lomustine (Systemic)
Loperamide (Oral)
Loratadine (Systemic)
Loratadine and Pseudoephedrine (Systemic)
Lorazepam (Systemic)
Losartan and Hydrochlorothiazide (Systemic)
Lovastatin (Systemic)

M

Mafenide (Topical)
Magnesium Hydroxide and Cascara Sagrada (Oral)
Magnesium Salicylate (Systemic)
Mangafodipir (Systemic)
Mazindol (Systemic)
Mechlorethamine (Systemic)

Mechlorethamine (Topical)
Meclizine (Systemic)
Meclofenamate (Systemic)
Medrogestone (Systemic)
Medroxyprogesterone (Systemic)
Mefloquine (Systemic)
Megestrol (Systemic)
Meloxicam (Systemic)
Melphalan (Systemic)
Menadiol (Systemic)
Mepenzolate (Systemic)
Mephobarbital (Systemic)
Meprobamate (Systemic)
Meprobamate and Aspirin (Systemic)
Mercaptopurine (Systemic)
Mesoridazine (Systemic)
Metformin (Systemic)
Methadone (Systemic)
Methantheline (Systemic)
Metharbital (Systemic)
Methazolamide (Systemic)
Methdilazine (Systemic)
Methicillin (Systemic)
Methimazole (Systemic).
Methotrexate-for cancer (Systemic)
Methotrexate-for noncancerous conditions (Systemic)
Methotrimeprazine (Systemic)
Methoxsalen (Extracorporeal-Systemic)
Methscopolamine (Systemic)
Methyclothiazide (Systemic)
Methyldopa (Systemic)
Methyldopa and Chlorothiazide (Systemic)
Methyldopa and Hydrochlorothiazide (Systemic)
Methylergonovine (Systemic)
Methylpredisolone (Systemic)
Methyltestosterone (Systemic)
Methysergide (Systemic)
Metoclopramide (Systemic)
Metolazone (Systemic)
Metoprolol (Systemic)
Metolazone (Systemic)
Metoprolol (Systemic)
Metoprolol and Hydrochlorothiazide (Systemic)

Metrizamide (Diagnostic)
Metronidazole (Systemic)
Metronidazole (Vaginal)
Metyrapone (Systemic)
Mexiletine (Systemic)
Mezlocillin (Systemic)
Midazolam (Systemic)
Minocycline (Systemic)
Minoxidil (Systemic)
Minoxidil (Topical)
Misoprostol (Systemic)
Mitomycin (Systemic)
Mitoxantrone (Systemic)
Mometasone (Topical)
Muromonab-CD3 (Systemic)
Mycophenolate (Systemic)

N

Nabilone (Systemic)
Nadolol (Systemic)
Nadolol and Bendroflumethiazide
    (Systemic)
Nafarelin (Systemic)
Nafcillin (Systemic)
Naftifine (Topical)
Nalidixic Acid (Systemic)
Nelfinavir (Systemic)
Nevirapine (Systemic)
Nicotine (Inhalation-Systemic)
Nicotine (Nasal)
Nicotine (Systemic)
Nisoldipine (Systemic)
Nitrazepam (Systemic)
Nitrofurantoin (Systemic)
Nitroglycerin-Topical (Systemic)
Nizatidine (Systemic)
Norethindrone (Systemic)
Norethindrone Acetate and Ethinyl
    Estradiol (Systemic)
Norethindrone and Ethinyl Estradiol
    (Systemic)
Norethindrone and Mestranol (Sys-
    temic)
Norfloxacin (Ophthalmic)
Norfloxacin (Systemic)
Norgestimate and 17 Beta-Estradiol
    (Systemic)

Norgestimate and Ethinyl Estradiol
    (Systemic)
Norgestrel and Ethinyl Estradiol
    (Systemic)
Nylidrin (Systemic)
Nystatin and Triamcinolone (Topical)

O

Ofloxacin (Otic)
Ofloxacin (Systemic)
Olanzapine (Systemic)
Olsalazine (Oral)
Omeprazole (Systemic)
Opium Tincture (Systemic)
Oxacillin (Systemic)
Oxazepam (Systemic)
Oxcarbazepine (Systemic)
Oxprenolol (Systemic)
Oxtriphylline (Systemic)
Oxtriphylline and Guaifenesin (Sys-
    temic)
Oxybutynin (Systemic)
Oxycodone and Aspirin (Systemic)
Oxytetracycline (Systemic)

P

Paclitaxel (Systemic)
Paregoric (Systemic)
Pegasparagase (Systemic)
Penbutolol (Systemic)
Penciclovir (Topical)
Penicillamine (Systemic)
Penicillin G (Systemic)
Penicillin V (Systemic)
Pentamidine (Systemic)
Pentazocine and Aspirin (Systemic)
Pentobarbital (Systemic)
Pentostatin (Systemic)
Pentoxifylline (Systemic)
Pergolide (Systemic)
Pericyazine (Systemic)
Permethrin (Topical)
Perphenazine (Systemic)
Perphenazine and Amitriptyline (Sys-
    temic)
Phendimetrazine (Systemic)

Phenindamine (Systemic)

Pheniramine, Codeine, and Guaifenesin (Systemic)

Pheniramine and Phenylephrine (Systemic)

Pheniramine, Phenylephrine, and Acetaminophen (Systemic)

Pheniramine, Phenylephrine, Codeine, Sodium Citrate, Sodium Salicylate, and Caffeine (Systemic)

Pheniramine, Phenylephrine, and Dextromethorphan (Systemic)

Pheniramine, Phenylephrine, Phenylpropanolamine, Hydrocodone, and Guaifenesin (Systemic)

Pheniramine, Phenylephrine, Sodium Salicylate, and Caffeine (Systemic)

Pheniramine, Phenyltoloxamine, Pyrilamine, and Phenylpropanolamine (Systemic)

Pheniramine, Pyrilamine, Hydrocodone, Potassium Citrate, and Ascorbic Acid (Systemic)

Pheniramine, Pyrilamine, Phenylephrine, Phenylpropanolamine, and Hydrocodone (Systemic)

Pheniramine, Pyrilamine, and Phenylpropanolamine (Systemic)

Pheniramine, Pyrilamine, Phenylpropanolamine, Acetaminophen, and Caffeine (Systemic)

Pheniramine, Pyrilamine, Phenylpropanolamine, and Codeine (Systemic)

Pheniramine, Pyrilamine, Phenylpropanolamine, and Dextromethorphan (Systemic)

Pheniramine, Pyrilamine, Phenylpropanolamine, Dextromethorphan, and Ammonium Chloride (Systemic)

Pheniramine, Pyrilamine, Phenylpropanolamine, and Hydrocodone (Systemic)

Pheniramine, Pyrilamine, Phenylpropanolamine, Hydrocodone, and Guaifenesin (Systemic)

Phenobarbital (Systemic)

Phenobarbital, Aspirin, and Codeine (Systemic)

Phentermine (Systemic)

Phenylbutazone (Systemic)

Phenylephrine and Codeine (Systemic)

Phenylephrine, Dextromethorphan, and Guaifenesin (Systemic)

Phenylephrine and Guaifenesin (Systemic)

Phenylephrine, Guaifenesin, Acetaminophen, Salicylamide, and Caffeine (Systemic)

Phenylephrine and Hydrocodone (Systemic)

Phenylephrine, Hydrocodone, and Guaifenesin (Systemic)

Phenylephrine, Phenylpropanolamine, Carbetapentane, and Potassium Guaiacolsulfonate (Systemic)

Phenylephrine, Phenylpropanolamine, and Guaifenesin (Systemic)

Phenylpropanolamine and Acetaminophen (Systemic)

Phenylpropanolamine, Acetaminophen, and Aspirin (Systemic)

Phenylpropanolamine, Acetaminophen, and Caffeine (Systemic)

Phenylpropanolamine, Acetaminophen, Salicylamide, and Caffeine (Systemic)

Phenylpropanolamine and Caramiphen (Systemic)

Phenylpropanolamine, Codeine, and Guaifenesin (Systemic)

Phenylpropanolamine and Dextromethorphan (Systemic)

Phenylpropanolamine, Dextromethorphan, and Acetaminophen (Systemic)

Phenylpropanolamine, Dextromethorphan, and Guaifenesin (Systemic)

Phenylpropanolamine, Dextromethorphan, Guaifenesin, and Acetaminophen (Systemic)

Phenylpropanolamine and
 Guaifenesin (Systemic)
Phenylpropanolamine and
 Hydrocodone (Systemic)
Phenylpropanolamine, Hydrocodone,
 Dextromethorphan, and Acetami-
 nophen (Systemic)
Phenyltoloaxamine and Hydrocodone
 (Systemic)
Phenyltoloxamine, Phenylpropanola-
 mine, and Acetaminophen (Sys-
 temic)
Phenytoin (Systemic)
Phytonadione (Systemic)
Pindolol (Systemic)
Pindolol and Hydrochlorothiazide
 (Systemic)
Pioglitazone (Systemic)
Piperacillin (Systemic)
Piperacillin and Tazobactam (Sys-
 temic)
Pipotiazine (Systemic)
Pirenzepine (Systemic)
Piroxicam (Systemic)
Pivampicillin (Systemic)
Pivmecillinam (Systemic)
Pneumococcal Conjugate Vaccine
 (Systemic)
Podofilox (Topical)
Polythiazide (Systemic)
Porfimer (Systemic)
Potassium Iodide (Systemic)
Pramipexole (Systemic)
Pravastatin (Systemic)
Prazepam (Systemic)
Praziquantel (Systemic)
Prazosin (Systemic)
Prazosin and Polythiazide (Systemic)
Prednisolone (Systemic)
Prednisone (Systemic)
Primidone (Systemic)
Probucol (Systemic)
Procarbazine (Systemic)
Prochlorperazine (Systemic)
Procyclidine (Systemic)
Progesterone (Systemic)
Promazine (Systemic)
Promethazine (Systemic)

Promethazine and Codeine (Systemic)
Promethazine, Codeine, and Potas-
 sium Guaiacolsulfonate (Sys-
 temic)
Promethazine and
 Dextromethorphan (Systemic)
Promethazine and Phenylephrine
 (Systemic)
Promethazine, Phenylephrine, and
 Codeine (Systemic)
Promethazine, Phenylephrine, Co-
 deine, and Potassium
 Guaiacolsulfonate (Systemic)
Promethazine, Phenylephrine, and
 Potassium Guaiacolsulfonate
 (Systemic)
Promethazine and Potassium
 Guaiacolsulfonate (Systemic)
Promethazine, Pseudoephedrine, and
 Dextromethorphan (Systemic)
Propafenone (Systemic)
Propantheline (Systemic)
Propoxyphene and Aspirin (Systemic)
Propoxyphene, Aspirin, and Caffeine
 (Systemic)
Propranolol (Systemic)
Propranolol and Hydrochlorothiazide
 (Systemic)
Propylthiouracil (Systemic)
Protirelin (Diagnostic)
Pseudoephedrine (Systemic)
Pseudoephedrine and Aspirin (Sys-
 temic)
Pseudoephedrine and Codeine (Sys-
 temic)
Pseudoephedrine, Codeine, and
 Guaifenesin (Systemic)
Pseudoephedrine and
 Dextromethorphan (Systemic)
Pseudoephedrine,
 Dextromethorphan, and Acetami-
 nophen (Systemic)
Pseudoephedrine,
 Dextromethorphan, and
 Guaifenesin (Systemic)
Pseudoephedrine,
 Dextromethorphan, Guaifenesin,
 and Acetaminophen (Systemic)

Pseudoephedrine and Guaifenesin (Systemic)

Pseudoephedrine and Hydrocodone (Systemic)

Pseudoephedrine, Hydrocodone, and Guaifenesin (Systemic)

Pseudoephedrine, Hydrocodone, and Potassium Guaiacolsulfonate (Systemic)

Pyrilamine and Codeine (Systemic)

Pyrilamine, Phenylephrine, Aspirin and Caffeine (Systemic)

Pyrilamine, Phenylephrine, and Codeine (Systemic)

Pyrilamine, Phenylephrine, and Dextromethorphan (Systemic)

Pyrilamine, Phenylephrine, and Hydrocodone (Systemic)

Pyrilamine, Phenylephrine, Hydrocodone, and Ammonium Chloride (Systemic)

Pyrilamine, Phenylpropanolamine, Acetaminophen, and Caffeine (Systemic)

Pyrilamine, Phenylpropanolamine, Dextromethorphan, Guaifenesin, potassium Citrate, and Citric Acid (Systemic)

Pyrilamine, Pseudoephedrine, Dextromethorphan, and Acetaminophen (Systemic)

Pyrimethamine (Systemic)

Q

Quazepam (Systemic)
Quetiapine (Systemic)
Quinethazone (Systemic)
Quinidine (Systemic)

R

Rabeprazole (Systemic)
Racepinephrine (Inhalation)
Radioiodinated Albumin (Diagnostic)
Raloxifene (Systemic)
Ranitidine (Systemic)
Ranitidine Bismuth Citrate (Systemic)

Rauwolfia Serpentina (Systemic)

Rauwolfia Serpentina and Bandroflumethiazide (Systemic)

Repaglinide (Systemic)

Reserpine (Systemic)

Reserpine and Chlorothiazide (Systemic)

Reserpine and Chlorthalidone (Systemic)

Reserpine, Hydralazine, and Hydrochlorothiazide (Systemic)

Reserpine and Hydrochlorothiazide (Systemic)

Reserpine and Hydroflumethiazide (Systemic)

Reserpine and Methyclothiazide (Systemic)

Reserpine and Polythiazide (Systemic)

Reserpine and Trichlormethiazide (Systemic)

Ribavirin (Systemic)

Rifampin and Isoniazid (Systemic)

Risedronate (Systemic)

Risperidone (Systemic)

Ritonavir (Systemic)

Rituximab (Systemic)

Rizatriptan (Systemic)

Rofecoxib (Systemic)

Ropinirole (Systemic)

Rosiglitazone (Systemic)

Rubidium Rb 82 (Diagnostic)

S

Salicylic Acid (Topical)
Salicylic Acid and Sulfur (Topical)
Salicylic Acid, Sulfur, and Coal Tar (Topical)
Salsalate (Systemic)
Samarium Sm 153 Lexidronam (Systemic)
Saquinavir (Systemic)
Scopolamine (Systemic)
Secobarbital (Systemic)
Secobarbital and Amobarbital (Systemic)
Silver Sulfadiazine (Topical)

Simvastatin (Systemic)
Sirolimus (Systemic)
Sodium Chromate Cr 51 (Diagnostic)
Sodium Fluoride F 18 (Diagnostic)
Sodium Iodide (Systemic)
Sodium Iodide I 123 (Diagnostic)
Sodium Iodide I 131 (Diagnostic)
Sodium iodide I 131 (Therapeutic)
Sodium Pertechnetale Tc 99m (Diagnostic)
Sodium Phosphate P 32 (Therapeutic)
Sodium Salicylate (Systemic)
Sotalol (Systemic)
Sparfloxacin (Systemic)
Spironolactone and Hydrochlorothiazide (Systemic)
Stavudine (Systemic)
Streptozocin (Systemic)
Strontium Chloride Sr 98 (Therapeutic)
Sulfadiazine (Systemic)
Sulfadiazine and Trimethoprim (Systemic)
Sulfadoxine and Pyrimethamine (Systemic)
Sulfamethizole (Systemic)
Sulfamethoxazole (Systemic)
Sulfamethoxazole and Phenazopyridine (Systemic)
Sulfamethoxazole and Trimethoprim (Systemic)
Sulfapyridine (Systemic)
Sulfasalazine (Systemic)
Sulfisoxazole (Systemic)
Sulfisoxazole and Phenazopyridine (Systemic)

T

Tacrine (Systemic)
Tacrolimus (Systemic)
Tamoxifen (Systemic)
Tazarotene (Topical)
Technetium Tc 99m Albumin (Diagnostic)
Technetium Tc 99m Albumin Aggregated (Diagnostic)
Technetium Tc 99m Albumin Colloid (Diagnostic)

Technetium Tc 99m Apcitide (Diagnostic)
Technetium Tc 99m Arcitumomab (Diagnostic)
Technetium Tc 99m Bicisate (Diagnostic)
Technetium Tc 99m Disofenin (Diagnostic)
Technetium Tc 99m Exametazime (Diagnostic)
Technetium Tc 99m Gluceptate (Diagnostic)
Technetium Tc 99m Lidofenin (Diagnostic)
Technetium Tc 99m Mebrofenin (Diagnostic)
Technetium Tc 99m Medronate (Diagnostic)
Technetium Tc 99m Mertiatide (Diagnostic)
Technetium Tc 99m Nofetumomab Merpentam (Diagnostic)
Technetium Tc 99m Oxidronate (Diagnostic)
Technetium Tc 99m Pentetate (Diagnostic)
Technetium Tc 99m Pyrophosphate (Diagnostic)
Technetium Tc 99m (Pyro- and trimeta-) Phosphates (Diagnostic)
Technetium Tc 99m Sestamibi (Diagnostic)
Technetium Tc 99m Succimer (Diagnostic)
Technetium Tc 99m Sulfur Colloid (Diagnostic)
Technetium Tc 99m Teboroxime (Diagnostic)
Technetium Tc 99m Tetrofosmin (Diagnostic)
Telmisartan (Systemic)
Temazepam (Systemic)
Temozolomide (Systemic)
Teniposide (Systemic)
Terazosin (Systemic)
Terbutaline (Inhalation)
Terbutaline (Oral/Injection)

Terfenadine (Systemic)
Testosterone (Systemic)
Testosterone and Estradiol (Systemic)
Tetracycline (Systemic)
Thalidomide (Systemic)
Thallous Chloride Tl 201 (Diagnostic)
Theophylline (Systemic)
Theophylline, Ephedrine, Guaifenesin, and Phenobarbital (Systemic)
Theophylline, Ephedrine, and Hydroxyzine (Systemic)
Theophylline, Ephedrine, and Phenobarbital (Systemic)
Theophylline and Guaifenesin (Systemic)
Thiabendazole (Systemic)
Thiethylperazine (Systemic)
Thioguanine (Systemic)
Thioproperazine (Systemic)
Thioridazine (Systemic)
Thiotepa (Systemic)
Thiothixene (Systemic)
Ticarcillin (Systemic)
Ticarcillin and Clavulanate (Systemic)
Timolol (Systemic)
Timolol and Hydrochlorothiazide (Systemic)
Tiopronin (Systemic)
Tixocortol (Rectal)
Tizanidine (Systemic)
Tobramycin and Dexamethasone (Ophthalmic)
Tolcapone (Systemic)
Tolterodine (Systemic)
Topotecan (Systemic)
Toremifene (Systemic)
Torsemide (Systemic)
Trandolapril and Verapamil (Systemic)
Trastuzumab (Systemic)
Tretinoin (Systemic)
Tretinoin (Topical)
Triamcinolone (Dental)
Triamcinolone (Systemic)
Triamcinolone (Topical)
Traimterene and Hydrochlorothiazide (Systemic)

Triazolam (Systemic)
Trichlormethiazide (Systemic)
Triclabendazole (Systemic)
Trifluoperazine (Systemic)
Triflupromazine (Systemic)
Trimethoprim (Systemic)
Trimetrexate (Systemic)
Tripelennamine (Systemic)
Triprolidine (Systemic)
Triprolidine and Pseudoephedrine (Systemic)
Triprolidine, Pseudoephedrine, and Codeine (Systemic)
Triprolidine, Pseudoephedrine, Codeine, and Guaifenesin (Systemic)
Triprolidine, Pseudoephedrine, and Dextromethorphan (Systemic)
Trovafloxacin (Systemic)
Tryopanoate (Diagnostic)

U

Uracil Mustard (Systemic)
Urofollitropin (Systemic)

V

Valacyclovir (Systemic)
Valproate Sodium (Systemic)
Valproic Acid (Systemic)
Valrubicin (Mucosal-Local)
Valsartan (Systemic)
Valsartan and Hydrochlorothiazide (Systemic)
Vinblastine (Systemic)
Vincrisine (Systemic)
Vinorelbine (Systemic)

W

Warfarin (Systemic)

X

Xenon Xe 127 (Diagnostic)
Xenon Xe 133 (Diagnostic)

Z

Zafirlukast (Systemic)
Zalcitabine (Systemic)
Zanamivir (Inhalation-Systemic)
Zidovudine (Systemic)
Zileuton (Systemic)
Zonisamide (Systemic)

Chapter 62

Breastfeeding and the Law

A Mother's Right to Breastfeed

Mothers have a right to breastfeed, and there is no law anywhere that we know of that prohibits breastfeeding or that tells a mother how long she can nurse. To the contrary, mothers have a constitutional right to breastfeed, as recognized by the U.S. Court of Appeals in *Dike v. Orange County School Board*, 650 F.2d 783 (5th Cir., 1981). In that case, a teacher wanted to nurse her baby on her duty-free lunch break. The school claimed that policies prohibited teachers from bringing their children onto school property, and also prohibited teachers from leaving the school grounds during the day. The trial court ruled that the mother had no right to breastfeed. In Dike, the appeals court reversed the case and remanded it for a new trial, stating that breastfeeding is a protected constitutional right.

"Breastfeeding is the most elemental form of parental care. It is a communion between mother and child that, like marriage, is 'intimate to the degree of being sacred,'" *Griswold v. Connecticut*, 381 U.S. at 486, 85 S. Ct. at 1682, 14 L. Ed. 2d at 516. "Nourishment is necessary to maintain the child's life, and the parent may choose to believe that breastfeeding will enhance the child's psychological as well as physical health. In light of the spectrum of interests that the Supreme

Excerpted from "A Brief Summary of Breastfeeding and the Law" by Elizabeth N. Baldwin, Esq. ©1995 La Leche League International (LLLI), www.laleche league.org; reprinted with permission. Reviewed and revised by David A. Cooke, M.D. on October 14, 2001.

Court has held specially protected, we conclude that the Constitution protects from excessive state interference a woman's decision respecting breastfeeding her child." 650 F.2d at 787.

The New Breastfeeding Legislation

State legislation tries to encourage breastfeeding by positively shifting the balance towards the right to breastfeed and away from other interests. Ten states have enacted legislation in the past three years that address a mother's right to breastfeed (see the section on current breastfeeding legislation). The purpose of this legislation is NOT to legalize it (it already is legal!) but to clarify this right, to encourage more mothers to breastfeed, and to help change the public perception that breastfeeding is indecent exposure.

Efforts at the Federal level have also been successful. The Right to Breastfeed Act (HR 1848) was signed into law in September 1999. This Act guarantees the right of any nursing mother and child authorized to be present in a federally-owned area to breastfeed without restriction. Additional legislation is currently under consideration in the U.S. Congress that explicitly state that breastfeeding is protected under Federal Civil Rights laws. Another bill has been introduced that provides tax incentives for businesses to provide breastfeeding-friendly workplaces.

As breastfeeding is not a lifestyle choice but a health choice for mother and baby, states are realizing that they can save money by encouraging breastfeeding, and that it will result in healthier mothers and babies.

Even if the mother's constitutional right to breastfeed doesn't apply in a situation (such as a private business), and the mother lives in a state that does not have this progressive legislation, her right to breastfeed is still protected. No one has the right to tell a mother how to feed her baby, or to discriminate against a woman because of her feeding choice.

As the legal system continues to recognize and encourage breastfeeding, a message is sent to the public at large that breastfeeding is an important issue—one that has an impact on our lives and the futures of our children. But society's views and taboos are not easily changed. Legislation that recognizes the importance of breastfeeding is just one step toward helping our society become more supportive of breastfeeding.

Types of Cases Involving Breastfeeding Issues

Nursing in Public

Mothers breastfeeding in public—such as in a restaurant, museum, library, or mall—may be told that they must stop. Most of the breastfeeding legislation deals with this issue, attempting to clarify that women have the right to breastfeed any place they have the right to be with their baby.

Employment Cases

Mothers seeking extended maternity leave, disability, or being prohibited from pumping or nursing at work comprise most of the employment cases. Recent legislation in two states attempts to encourage mothers to continue breastfeeding when they return to work.

Jury Duty

Breastfeeding mothers can be called for jury duty. The separations necessary to serve on a jury may pose an undue burden on the breastfeeding mother and child. One state has specifically excluded breastfeeding mothers from jury duty.

Family Law Cases

Most breastfeeding cases are family law, divorce, or paternity, where the father seeks custody or lengthy visitation with a baby or nursing child. Occasionally the mother may be defending her choice to breastfeed, such as with extended breastfeeding.

Social Service Agency or Criminal Cases

A small number of cases involve breastfeeding mothers being reported to a social service agency for abuse or neglect. Occasionally the allegations against the mother may involve breastfeeding issues like extended breastfeeding or low weight gain. Note that breastfeeding is not abuse or neglect, and no court has found so. Most of these cases involve a mother accused of abuse/neglect for issues other than breastfeeding, whose breastfeeding relationship may be jeopardized by separations from her child. Criminal cases can involve prosecution for drugs and breastfeeding, or just involve a breastfeeding mother sentenced to prison.

Civil Cases

Personal injury cases can involve breastfeeding issues, such as when a mother's breast is damaged in an accident, or where injury to the mother results in weaning of the baby.

Nursing in Public

Over the past few years, much publicity has been given to mothers who are told to stop breastfeeding in public. Mothers in some malls, museums, libraries and stores have been told that their breastfeeding is indecent and not allowed. Most of these situations are easily resolved by educating those involved about the importance of breastfeeding and a woman's right to breastfeed where she has the right to be.

Many of the mothers who are told to stop breastfeeding are new mothers who never nursed in public before. By trying to be so discreet, they may call attention to themselves. A mother insuring that nothing shows may turn the chair around, or put a shawl over her shoulder. Although none of her breast or nipple shows, everyone knows what she is doing. The more experienced nursers are often not noticed, as they have learned to nurse discretely without anyone knowing that they are breastfeeding. The new mother who is told to stop nursing in public may be very humiliated and embarrassed. There is a greater chance that the less experienced breastfeeding mother will choose to wean or to give bottles in public in order to avoid going through such an experience again. Some pregnant mothers may choose not to breastfeed just because she might have to deal with a situation like this.

The breastfeeding legislation that has been enacted in the United States over the past few years typically clarifies the fact that breastfeeding is not indecent exposure, and thus not criminal behavior. Most of the states have gone further than this, and have made it perfectly clear that a woman has a right to breastfeed any place she has the right to be, even if the mother's nipple is exposed during or incidental to breastfeeding. New York has gone furthest, in that mothers are provided with a remedy if they are prevented from breastfeeding. New York's law protects the right to breastfeed in public as a mother's civil right! It is hoped that enacting legislation guaranteeing the right to breastfeed in public will help to remove just one more stumbling block from a mother's decision to breastfeed or continue breastfeeding.

Society is slowly changing its attitudes about breastfeeding. We know that breastfeeding reduces both the mother's and baby's risk of serious illnesses. And we know that if mothers don't nurse on demand or give bottles in the early weeks, that breastfeeding can be jeopardized. Would we want even one mother or one baby to have an increased risk of illness just because someone didn't want to see it? It is for these reasons that legislation is being enacted to specifically clarify a mother's right to breastfeed in public.

Mothers who are told to stop breastfeeding can let the person know that they have the right to feed their baby in this healthy way. They can also let the establishment know that these types of attitudes are precisely why so many states have clarified their laws to make it perfectly clear that mothers can breastfeed anywhere they have a right to be. If a mother is in a state with current legislation, she can let them know what the law says.

Employment Cases

As more women learn that it is not only possible, but often very beneficial to the baby and mother to continue breastfeeding when they return to work, more situations evolve where mothers are not supported by their employers. Some mothers are not given sufficient time to pump. Many of these situations are resolved easily by educating the employer. Mothers need to keep their anger out of it and approach the employer in a friendly, helpful way.

The trend is for employers to support breastfeeding since a healthier baby results in the mother missing less time from work. Over the past few years, more and more companies have installed breast pump rooms and looked at how the mother's schedule can be arranged to provide sufficient time to pump.

Mothers looking for assistance in one of these situations may want to first determine if there are any employee advocates, such as the human resources department or a union. Mothers should get legal advice immediately from a labor law attorney in her area so as to determine what time limits may apply to her situation. This is imperative if there is any chance that there may be repercussions from her decision to continue breastfeeding, as there are strict time limits on filing discrimination claims. If missed, this could result in the mother having no legal recourse. Many employment situations may have discrimination issues which are either directly or indirectly related to breastfeeding.

Jury Duty

Some states exclude women at home with young children, but others don't. Educating is your first step. A doctor's note may be a second. In some situations, explaining the situation to the judge may be necessary.

Family Law Cases

The courts are clear that they will not pick breastfeeding over a bond with the father. Breastfeeding is protected in family law cases by showing the court how the father can have a bond, while breastfeeding is protected.

The reason is that the primary goal of the courts is to find a way for the child to have a bond with both parents after they separate. Although the mother's bond is born of biology, the father's bond is just as important. Many courts look at which parent will provide better access to the other parent with the child, and encourage their bond, in looking at who should get custody.

Thus, to protect breastfeeding, mothers generally do better if they show the court how the father's bond can be promoted. For instance, short, frequent visits with the father can help accomplish this goal with infants. Visits should gradually increase in length as the child grows.

Preparing realistic, practical visitation plans that start out with significant visitation with the father and work up to weekends or what the father wants is a good way to convince a judge that the breastfeeding relationship can be protected while the father's bond is promoted.

In many cases, breastfeeding is intertwined with separation issues. For instance, if a mother proves the superiority of breastmilk but fails to touch on separation issues, she may be told to pump her breasts for lengthy separations. Rarely will a judge tell a mother to wean; in most cases breastfeeding is affected indirectly as a result of the separation. Most cases require the testimony of psychiatrists or psychologists to address the issue of what effect lengthy separations can have on the child.

Parents have a difficult road ahead of them if they are trying to restrict the other parent's contact on the grounds of abuse. Courts want the child to have a bond with both parents. The goals in protecting the breastfeeding relationship and protecting a party from abuse are often inconsistent with each other. With breastfeeding issues, one is more likely to be trying to reshape rather than restrict time with the other parent, avoiding lengthy separations with frequent and continuing contact. When a party alleges abuse, the court may be primarily concerned with how to keep the contact between the parents to a bare minimum, which often results in more lengthy separations and less frequent visits.

Keep in mind that the best way to protect the breastfeeding relationship is to work things out with the baby's father. It is almost unheard of for a judge to put off overnight visitation past age two, and yet many mothers accomplish this by settling their cases. There are so many ways to settle a case—with lawyers, without, through mediation, etc. Parents can discuss with their lawyer the various ways that cases are settled.

Criminal and Social Service Cases

Although several social service agencies have addressed the issue of extended breastfeeding, none have found it to be abuse or neglect. Cases in the United States have dealt with the issue of breastfeeding as long as age six, seven, or even eight years. Most are resolved easily by providing information on the normalcy of extended breastfeeding.

The large majority of social service agency cases do not involve breastfeeding issues directly, but rather involve a breastfeeding mother accused of abuse or neglect for non-breastfeeding matters. In that case, the effect of lengthy separations can result in abrupt weaning, or even severance of the parent's bond with the child. It is important to educate on these psychological issues, and help find acceptable alternatives to placement while the case is being investigated.

Any person reported for abuse needs to take it very seriously, as decisions can affect the entire parent/child relationship. It is important to seek competent legal advice before volunteering information or agreeing to supervision.

Another breastfeeding issue that has arisen in the social service agencies is that of low weight gain, or failure to thrive. Although these cases are rare, some jurisdictions may closely scrutinize situations where the baby is below the 10th percentile.

Rarely is breastfeeding raised directly in criminal cases. An exception is the prosecution of mothers for breastfeeding while doing illegal drugs. Criminal cases usually involve a breastfeeding mother sentenced to jail time. Courts generally hold that constitutional rights, and especially the right to rear our children, are incompatible with prison. However, some places may have special programs for mothers and newborns to have contact, and some judges have delayed sentencing to allow the mother to wean.

Civil Cases

There have been some lawsuits by breastfeeding mothers for damages for either the breastfeeding relationship failing because of the accident, or where the mother seeks damages for injury to her breast.

In one case, an arbitrator awarded a mother one year's worth of formula for an accident which contributed to (but did not cause) the breastfeeding failure!

References

1. Baldwin EN: Handling legal calls. *Leaven* Nov/Dec1994;30(6).

2. Baldwin EN, Friedman KA: Breastfeeding and visitation. *New Beginnings* Jan/Feb 1996;13(1).

3. Baldwin EN, Friedman KA: Breastfeeding legislation in the United States. *New Beginnings* Nov/Dec 1994.

4. Baldwin EN: You can't call me for jury duty, I'm breastfeeding. *Leaven* Sept/Oct 1994;30(5).

5. Baldwin EN, Friedman KA: So I nursed every forty-five minutes. *Mothering* Spring 1994.

6. Baldwin EN, Friedman KA: Is breastfeeding really a visitation issue? *Mothering* Fall 1993;68.

7. Baldwin EN: Extended breastfeeding and the law. *Mothering* Spring 1993;66.

8. Baldwin EN: So, is it against the law to breastfeed? *Leaven* Mar/April 1996;28(2).

9. Grant JP: Call to physicians for support. *Baby-Friendly Hospital Initiative Newsletter* Jul/Aug 1994 (available from LLLI).

10. Kneidel S: Nursing beyond one year. *New Beginnings* Jul/Aug 1990.

11. La Leche League International: *Breastfeeding does make a difference*. Publication No. 64.

12. La Leche League International: 1995: *Facts about breastfeeding*. Publication No. 545g.

13. La Leche League International: *Women, working, and breastfeeding*. Publication No. 432b.

14. Suhler A, Bornmann PG, Scott JW: The lactation consultant as an expert witness. *J Human Lactation* September 1991;7(3).

15. Wilson-Clay B: Extended breastfeeding as a legal issue: An annotated bibliography. *J Human Lactation* June 1990;6(2).

Chapter 63

Government Initiatives to Increase Breastfeeding Rates

Breastfeeding as a Public Health Challenge

Recognizing the considerable scientific evidence that states breastfeeding is one of the most important contributors to infant health, the Office of the U.S. Surgeon General released the first comprehensive national framework to promote breastfeeding and optimal breastfeeding practices. The Health and Human Services (HHS) *Blueprint for Action on Breastfeeding* was developed by health and scientific experts from fourteen federal agencies and twenty-three health care professional organizations, including the American Academy of Pediatrics and the American Academy of Family Physicians.

During the past fifteen years, the Office of the Surgeon General has highlighted the public health importance of breastfeeding through numerous workshops and publications. Scientific evidence suggests that breastfeeding provides a range of benefits for an infant's growth, immunity, and development. In addition, breastfeeding has also been shown to improve maternal health.

Scientific evidence states that human milk contains an abundance of factors that are active against infection. Breastfed infants, compared with formula-fed infants, produce enhanced immune responses

Office of the U.S. Surgeon General Press Release, October 30, 2000. "Surgeon General Releases First Comprehensive Framework to Increase Breastfeeding Rates and Promote Optimal Breastfeeding Practices." Excerpts of the Department of Health and Human Services "Blueprint for Action on Breastfeeding." Both documents available at www.4woman.gov.

to polio, tetanus, diphtheria, and common respiratory infections. Recent research also suggests that breastfeeding reduces the risk of chronic diseases among children, including diabetes, inflammatory bowel disease, allergies and asthma, and childhood cancer.

Mothers also experience benefits from breastfeeding, including less postpartum bleeding, earlier return to pre-pregnancy weight, a possible reduced risk of ovarian cancer and premenopausal breast cancer, and positive hormonal, physical and psychosocial effects. The Blueprint recommends that mothers with certain conditions, including Hepatitis C, substance abuse problems, some environmental exposures, metabolic disorders, and breast implants should check with their doctor before breastfeeding. Women with HIV/ AIDS and human T-cell leukemia virus type 1 (HTLV-1) should not breastfeed.

Despite the many benefits of breastfeeding, statistics reveal that 64 percent of American mothers breastfeed in the early postpartum period, with only 29 percent still breastfeeding six months after birth. Racial and ethnic disparities in breastfeeding are wide, revealing extremely low rates among African-American women.

"Low breastfeeding rates documented in the Blueprint for Action are a serious public health challenge, particularly in certain minority communities," said David Satcher, M.D., U.S. Surgeon General and Assistant Secretary for Health. "With scientific evidence indicating that breastfeeding can play an important role in an infant's health, the time has come for us to work together to promote optimal breastfeeding practices. Each of us, at all levels of the public and private sectors, must now turn these recommendations into programs that best suit the needs of our own communities."

Increasing Breastfeeding Rates in the United States: A Strategic Plan

Healthy People 2010, the nation's health agenda for the next decade, has set an objective to increase the proportion of all mothers who breastfeed in the early postpartum period to 75 percent. "The Healthy People objectives will be realized only when we work together to put in place culturally appropriate strategies to promote breastfeeding, with particular emphasis on education and support from health care professionals, employers and family members, especially fathers and grandmothers," said Wanda Jones, Dr.P.H., Deputy Assistant Secretary for Health (Women's Health) and director of the Office on Women's Health.

The Blueprint for Action promotes a plan for breastfeeding based on education, training, awareness, support, and research. Specifically, the plan lays out a framework based on the recommendation that infants be exclusively breastfed during the first four to six months of life, preferably for a full six months. The plan also suggests that, ideally, breastfeeding should continue through the first year of life.

The Blueprint offers action steps for the health care system, families, the community, researchers, and the workplace, to better focus attention on the importance of breastfeeding. It recommends that health care professionals who provide maternal and child care are trained on the basics of lactation and breastfeeding counseling, that women who return to work after childbirth should have access to child care facilities or private rooms on site to accommodate breastfeeding, that social support and information resources be established for women such as hotlines and peer counseling, and that research be conducted on issues surrounding breastfeeding.

Goal 1: Assure access to comprehensive, current, and culturally appropriate lactation care and services for all women, children, and families.

- **Objective 1.1:** Identify and disseminate evidence-based best practices and policies throughout the health care system.

- **Objective 1.2:** Educate all health care providers and payers regarding appropriate breastfeeding and lactation support.

- **Objective 1.3:** Ensure that all women have access to appropriate breastfeeding support within the family and/or community.

- **Objective 1.4:** Ensure the routine collection and coordination of breastfeeding data by federal, state, and local governments and other organizations; foster additional research of breastfeeding.

Goal 2: Ensure that breastfeeding is recognized as the normal and preferred method of feeding infants and young children.

- **Objective 2.1:** Develop a positive and desirable image of breastfeeding for the American public.

- **Objective 2.2:** Reduce the barriers to breastfeeding posed by the marketing of breastmilk substitutes.

Goal 3: Ensure that all Federal, State, and local laws relating to child welfare and family law recognize and support the importance and practice of breastfeeding.

- **Objective 3.1:** Ensure that all lawmakers and government officials at Federal, State, and local levels are aware of the importance of protecting, promoting, and supporting breastfeeding.

Goal 4: Increase protection, promotion, and support for breastfeeding mothers in the work force.

- **Objective 4.1:** The rights of women in the workplace will be recognized in public and private sectors.

- **Objective 4.2:** Ensure that all mothers are able to seamlessly integrate breastfeeding and employment.

The Blueprint was developed by the Subcommittee on Breastfeeding, under the auspices of the HHS Environmental Health Policy Committee, including members of the Federal Interagency Working Group on Women's Health and the Environment, coordinated by the Office on Women's Health.

The full text of the HHS Blueprint for Action on Breastfeeding can be found on a new specialty section on breastfeeding on the Web site of the National Women's Health Information Center (www.4woman.gov) or through its toll-free telephone service at 1-800-994-WOMAN (TDD: 1-888-220-5446).

Chapter 64

Breastfeeding Resources

Organizations That Offer Support

Human Milk Banking Association of North America
c/o Mothers' Milk Bank
3000 New Bern Ave.
Raleigh, NC 27610
Phone: 919-350-8599
Website: www.hmbana.org

The Human Milk Banking Association of North America, Inc. is a nonprofit organization established in 1985. Some of its activities include annually reviewing and revising guidelines for donor human milk banking practices in North America to assure a safe, nutritious product; providing a forum for information sharing among experts on human milk and lactation related to human milk banking; and facilitating communication among member banks to assure adequate distribution of donor milk to patients in all parts of North America.

International Lactation Consultant Association
1500 Sunday Dr.
Raleigh, NC 27607
Phone: 919-787-5181
Fax: 919-787-4916
Website: www.ilca.org
E-mail: ilca@erols.com

ILCA promotes the professional development, advancement, and recognition of lactation consultants worldwide for the benefit of breastfeeding women, infants, and children. This organization can refer you to a lactation consultant who has been board certified as a health care provider.

La Leche League International
1400 N. Meacham Rd.
P.O. Box 4079
Schaumburg, IL 60168-4079
Phone: 847-519-7730
Fax: 847-519-0035
Website: www.lalecheleague.org
Email: LLLHQ@llli.org

La Leche League is dedicated to providing education, information, support, and encouragement to women who want to breastfeed. Website includes frequently asked questions, links to breastfeeding resources, an on-line catalog, and a national directory of La Leche League groups.

Nursing Mother's Counsel, Inc.
P.O. Box 50063
Palo Alto, CA 94303
Phone: 415-386-2229
Website: www.nursingmothers.org
E-mail: nmc@best.com

NMC is a non-affiliated, non-profit organization whose goal is to help mothers enjoy a relaxed and happy feeding relationship with their babies by providing breastfeeding information and support. Most help can be provided over the telephone, but the NMC also offers home visits to resolve difficult problems. NMC services are provided without fee or obligation.

Postpartum Support International
927 N. Kellogg
Santa Barbara, CA 93111
- Phone: 805-967-7636
Fax: 805-967-0608
Website: www.iup.edu/anthropology/postpartum

Postpartum Education for Parents

P.O. Box 6154
Santa Barbara, CA 93160
Phone: 408-774-1464
Website: www.sbpep.org
E-mail: pepmail@yahoo.com

Women, Infants, and Children (WIC) Program

United States Department of Agriculture
Supplemental Food Program Division
Food and Nutrition Services, USDA
3101 Park Center Dr., 5th
Alexandria, VA 22302
Toll Free: 888-942-3678
Phone: 703-305-2746
Fax: 703-305-2196
Website: http://www.fns.usda.gov/wic

The WIC program mission is to safeguard the health of low-income women, infants, and children up to age 5 who are at nutritional risk by providing nutritious foods to supplement diets, information on healthy eating, and referrals to health care. The WIC website is maintained by the Food and Nutrition Service (FNS), a federal agency of the U.S. Department of Agriculture, who is responsible for administering the WIC Program at the national and regional levels. See website to find listings of the toll-free numbers of WIC state agencies.

For Further Reading

American Academy of Pediatrics Policy Statement on Breastfeeding

Website: www.aap.org/policy/re9729.html

This document summarizes the benefits of breastfeeding to the infant, the mother, and the nation, and sets forth principles to guide the pediatrician and other health care providers in the initiation and maintenance of breastfeeding. The policy statement also delineates the various ways in which pediatricians can promote, protect, and support breastfeeding, not only in their individual practices but also in the hospital, medical school, community, and nation.

343

Health Education Associates Breastfeeding Pamphlets
8 Jan Sebastian Way #13
Sandwich, MA 02563-2354
Phone: 888-888-8077
Fax: 508-888-8050
Website: www.healthed.cc
E-mail: hea@capecod.net

Many titles are available, including, "Sleep Patterns of Breastfed Babies," "If Your Grandchild is Breastfed," and "How to Nurse Modestly." See full list of titles online.

New Beginnings Magazine
1400 N. Meacham Rd.
P.O. Box 4079
Schaumburg, IL 60168-4079
Phone: 847-519-7730
Fax: 847-519-0035
Website: www.lalecheleague.org

La Leche League's breastfeeding journal, published bimonthly and available with LLLI membership. This magazine is filled with stories, hints, and inspiration from other breastfeeding families.

Breastfeeding Books

Behan, Eileen. *Eat Well, Lose Weight While Breastfeeding: the Complete Nutrition Book for Nursing Mothers*, Random House Inc., 1992.

Bumgarner, Norma J. *Mothering Your Nursing Toddler*, Schamburg, IL: La Leche League International, 1982.

Gotsch, Gwen. *Breastfeeding Pure and Simple*, Schamburg, IL: La Leche League International, 1994.

Gotsch, Gwen. *Breastfeeding Your Premature Baby*, Schamburg, IL: La Leche League International, 1999.

Granju, Katie Allison and Kennedy, Betsy. *Attachment Parenting: Instinctive Care for Your Baby and Young Child*, New York: Pocket Books, 1999.

Gromada, Karen Kerkhoff. *Mothering Multiples: Breastfeeding and Caring for Twins or More*, Schamburg, IL: La Leche League International, 1999.

Huggins, Kathleen. *The Nursing Mother's Companion*, Boston: Harvard Common Press, 1995.

Kitzinger, Sheila. *Breastfeeding Your Baby*, New York: Knopf, 1998.

La Leche League International. *The Womanly Art of Breastfeeding*, Schaumburg, IL: La Leche League International, 1992.

Newman, Jack and Pitman, Teresa. *The Ultimate Breastfeeding Book of Answers: The Most Comprehensive Problem-Solution Guide to Breastfeeding from the Foremost Experts in North America*, Prima Communications, Inc., 2000.

Pryor, Gale. *Nursing Mother, Working Mother: The Essential Guide for Breastfeeding and Staying Close to Your Baby After You Return to Work*. Boston: Harvard Common Press, 1997.

Sears, William and Sears, Martha. *The Breastfeeding Book: Everything You Need to Know About Nursing Your Child from Birth through Weaning*, Boston: Little, Brown and Co. 2000.

Tamaro-Natt, Janet. *So That's What They're For: Breastfeeding Basics*, Holsbrook, MA: Adams Media, 1998.

West, Diana. Defining Your Own Success: *Breastfeeding after Breast Reduction Surgery*, Schamburg, IL: La Leche League International, 2001.

Websites with Breastfeeding Information

Breastfeeding.Com
Website: www.breastfeeding.com
E-mail: feedback@breastfeeding.com

Comprehensive website featuring breastfeeding information, advocacy, humor, support, and resources. Includes a national directory of lactation consultants and video clips of hunger cues and positioning.

The Christian Parent's Guide to Breastfeeding
Website: www.christianparent.com
E-Mail: info@christianparent.com

Explores the spiritual value in nourishing and nurturing your children according to God's plan, and studies references to nursing in Scripture.

LactNews OnLine
Website: http://www.jump.net/~bwc

Provides breastfeeding advocates with information about breast-feeding courses, conferences, and educational materials.

National Women's Health Information Center, United States Department of Health and Human Services
8550 Arlington Blvd., Suite 300
Fairfax, VA 22031
Phone: 800-994-9662; Fax: 703-560-6598; TDD: 888-220-5446
Website: www.4woman.gov/Breastfeeding/index.htm
E-mail: 4women@soza.com

Read the 2000 *Blueprint for Action on Breastfeeding* online.

Promotion of Mother's Milk, Inc. (ProMoM)
P.O. Box 3912
New York, NY 10163
Website: www.promom.org

Promotion of Mother's Milk (ProMoM) is dedicated to increasing public awareness and public acceptance of breastfeeding. Website contains activism opportunities; articles; message boards; a comprehensive list of breastfeeding links; and lists of pro-breastfeeding doctors, hospitals, and businesses. Also includes a large selection of Dr. Jack Newman's articles.

Pumping Moms Information Exchange
Website: www.pumpingmoms.org
E-mail: listowner@pumpingmoms.org

Provides information as support for moms who are expressing milk for their children. Read frequently asked questions, find useful links, and subscribe to the e-mail list discussing pumping and related topics.

San Diego County Breastfeeding Coalition
c/o Children's Hospital and Health Center
3020 Children's Way, MC 5073
San Diego, CA 92123-4282
Website: www.breastfeeding.org
E-mail: sdbc@breastfeeding.org

A non-profit association of health care professionals whose mission is to promote and support breastfeeding through education and outreach in the community. Website contains a large variety of articles and links, and is a resource for the public as well as health care professionals.

Breastfeeding Products and Supplies

Elizabeth Lee Designs
P.O. Box 696
Bluebell, UT 84007
Toll Free: 800-449 3350
Phone: 435-353-4344
Website: www.elizabethlee.com

Offers patterns for sewing nursing clothes and baby items.

Medela, Inc.
P.O. Box 660
McHenry, IL 60051-0660
Phone: 800-435-8316; Fax: 815-363-9941
Website: www.medela.com
E-Mail: customer.service@medela.com

Medela provides breast pumps and breastfeeding accessories to nursing mothers and health care facilities in the United States. Medela has also developed a workplace program to meet the needs of working mothers. Through the Corporate Lactation Program, businesses support breastfeeding employees and their families by providing breastfeeding counseling and breast pumps in an accessible, private, pleasant location.

Motherhood Nursingwear
Phone: 800-4MOM2BE
Website: www.motherhoodnursing.com
E-Mail: info@motherhoodnursing.com

Large assortment of quality nursing clothes at low prices. Find a store in your area or order on-line.

The Motherwear Catalog
Phone: 800-950-2500
E-mail: customerservice@motherwear.com
Website: www.motherwear.com

Motherwear offers a large selection of nursing clothes and bras, as well as breastfeeding products and information.

Nursing Mothers Supplies

Phone: 800-688-6545

Website: www.nursingmothersupplies.com

Offers breast pumps, nursing aids, nursing pads, maternity products, and nursing bras. A breastfeeding counselor is available to help with pumping questions.

Index

Index

351

M

mafenide 320
magnesium hydroxide 320
magnesium salicylate 320
malocclusion 5
mammary gland, defined 308
mangafodipir 320
mastitis
  defined 308
  described 51, *155*, 161–65, 299
"Mastitis" (Sears) 161n
maternal health, breastfeeding 36,
  297–301, 337–38
maternity leave, legislation 331
mazindol 320
mechlorethamine 320
meclizine 320
meclofenamate 320
meconium 108–9
Medela, Inc., contact information 347
medical professionals
  breastfeeding education 64–66
  breastfeeding knowledge 16–17
  breastfeeding support 81–84
  see also lactation professionals
The Medical Reporter 3n
medications
  breastfeeding 27, 52, 98, 297–98
  human immunodeficiency virus
    289–90
  international travel 132
  see also *individual medications*
medrogestone 320
medroxyprogesterone 320
mefloquine 320
megestrol 320
meloxicam 320
melphalan 320
menadiol 320
menopause, breastfeeding 29
mepenzolate 320
mephobarbital 320
meprobamate 320
mercaptopurine 320
mesoridazine 320
metformin 320
methadone 320

methantheline 320
metharbital 320
methazolamide 320
methdilazine 320
methicillin 320
methimazole 320
methotrexate 320
methotrimeprazine 320
methoxsalen 320
methscopolamine 320
methyclothiazide 320
methyldopa 320
methylergonovine 320
methylpredisolone 320
methyltestosterone 320
methysergide 320
metoclopramide 183–85, 320
metolazone 320
metoprolol 320
metrizamide 321
metronidazole 298, 321
metyrapone 321
mexiletine 321
mezlocillin 321
MICROMEDEX Thompson Health-
  care, medications publication 311n
midazolam 321
milk ducts, clogged 51, *155*, 159–61
milk ejection reflex (letdown)
  defined 308
  described 56
milk production, described 59–62
milk supply, defined 308
minocycline 321
minoxidil 321
misoprostol 321
mitomycin 321
mitoxantrone 321
"Moderate Weight Loss OK for Overweight Moms Who Breast Feed"
  (NICHD) 139n
mometasone 321
Morhrbacher, Nancy 203n
Motherhood Nursingwear, Web site
  information 347
Mothers' Milk Bank (Austin, TX) 263n
  contact information 266
Mother's Milk Bank, P/SL Medical
  Center, contact information 265

V

valacyclovir 326
valproate sodium 326
valproic acid 326
valrubicin 326
valsartan 326
vinblastine 326
vincrisine 326
vinorelbine 326
Vinther, Tine Dige 59n
vitamin supplements, breastfeeding 26–27, 117–18
vomiting, defined 310

W

warfarin 298, 326
weaning
    age recommendations 69, 133–34
    defined 310
    pregnancy 22
weight loss, breastfeeding 7, 26, 96–97, 135, 139–41
wet nurses 29
"Why Breastfeed?" 283n
"WIC Infant Feeding Practices Study: Breastfeeding Duration, Attitudes and Practices" (USDA) 41m
WIC Program *see* Women, Infants, and Children Program
WideSmiles, publications 251n
Williams, Rebecca D. 47n
Wilmington Mothers' Milk Bank, Medical Center of Delaware, contact information 265
The Womanly Art of Breastfeeding (LLLI) 117

Women, Infants, and Children Program (WIC)
    breastfeeding statistics 42–44
    contact information 343
"Work and Continue to Breastfeed" (San Diego County Breastfeeding Coalition) 219n
workplace issues
    breastfeeding 8–9, 18, 24, 51–52, 219–24
    breast pumping 222, 333
World Health Organization (WHO)
    formula company marketing practices 16
    publications 59n, 305n

X

xenon 326

Y

yeast infections 204
"You Can Still Breastfeed" (Newman) 297n

Z

zafirlukast 327
zalcitabine 327
zanamivir 327
Zeretzke, Karen 193n
zidovudine 327
zileuton 327
Zoloft (sertraline) 298
zonisamide 327

Health Reference Series
COMPLETE CATALOG

Adolescent Health Sourcebook

Basic Consumer Health Information about Common Medical, Mental, and Emotional Concerns in Adolescents, Including Facts about Acne, Body Piercing, Mononucleosis, Nutrition, Eating Disorders, Stress, Depression, Behavior Problems, Peer Pressure, Violence, Gangs, Drug Use, Puberty, Sexuality, Pregnancy, Learning Disabilities, and More

Along with a Glossary of Terms and Other Resources for Further Help and Information

Edited by Chad T. Kimball. 658 pages. 2002. 0-7808-0248-9. $78.

■

AIDS Sourcebook, 1st Edition

Basic Information about AIDS and HIV Infection, Featuring Historical and Statistical Data, Current Research, Prevention, and Other Special Topics of Interest for Persons Living with AIDS

Along with Source Listings for Further Assistance

Edited by Karen Bellenir and Peter D. Dresser. 831 pages. 1995. 0-7808-0031-1. $78.

"One strength of this book is its practical emphasis. The intended audience is the lay reader . . . useful as an educational tool for health care providers who work with AIDS patients. Recommended for public libraries as well as hospital or academic libraries that collect consumer materials."
— Bulletin of the Medical Library Association, Jan '96

"This is the most comprehensive volume of its kind on an important medical topic. Highly recommended for all libraries."
— Reference Book Review, '96

"Very useful reference for all libraries."
— Choice, Association of College and Research Libraries, Oct '95

"There is a wealth of information here that can provide much educational assistance. It is a must book for all libraries and should be on the desk of each and every congressional leader. Highly recommended."
— AIDS Book Review Journal, Aug '95

"Recommended for most collections."
— Library Journal, Jul '95

■

AIDS Sourcebook, 2nd Edition

Basic Consumer Health Information about Acquired Immune Deficiency Syndrome (AIDS) and Human Immunodeficiency Virus (HIV) Infection, Featuring Updated Statistical Data, Reports on Recent Research and Prevention Initiatives, and Other Special Topics of Interest for Persons Living with AIDS, Including New Antiretroviral Treatment Options, Strategies for Combating Opportunistic Infections, Information about Clinical Trials, and More

Along with a Glossary of Important Terms and Resource Listings for Further Help and Information

Edited by Karen Bellenir. 751 pages. 1999. 0-7808-0225-X. $78.

"Highly recommended."
— American Reference Books Annual, 2000

"Excellent sourcebook. This continues to be a highly recommended book. There is no other book that provides as much information as this book provides."
— AIDS Book Review Journal, Dec-Jan 2000

"Recommended reference source."
— Booklist, American Library Association, Dec '99

"A solid text for college-level health libraries."
— The Bookwatch, Aug '99

Cited in Reference Sources for Small and Medium-Sized Libraries, American Library Association, 1999

■

Alcoholism Sourcebook

Basic Consumer Health Information about the Physical and Mental Consequences of Alcohol Abuse, Including Liver Disease, Pancreatitis, Wernicke-Korsakoff Syndrome (Alcoholic Dementia), Fetal Alcohol Syndrome, Heart Disease, Kidney Disorders, Gastrointestinal Problems, and Immune System Compromise and Featuring Facts about Addiction, Detoxification, Alcohol Withdrawal, Recovery, and the Maintenance of Sobriety

Along with a Glossary and Directories of Resources for Further Help and Information

Edited by Karen Bellenir. 613 pages. 2000. 0-7808-0325-6. $78.

"This title is one of the few reference works on alcoholism for general readers. For some readers this will be a welcome complement to the many self-help books on the market. Recommended for collections serving general readers and consumer health collections."
— E-Streams, Mar '01

"This book is an excellent choice for public and academic libraries."
— American Reference Books Annual, 2001

"Recommended reference source."
— Booklist, American Library Association, Dec '00

"Presents a wealth of information on alcohol use and abuse and its effects on the body and mind, treatment, and prevention."
— SciTech Book News, Dec '00

"Important new health guide which packs in the latest consumer information about the problems of alcoholism."
— Reviewer's Bookwatch, Nov '00

SEE ALSO Drug Abuse Sourcebook, Substance Abuse Sourcebook

Allergies Sourcebook, 1st Edition

Basic Information about Major Forms and Mechanisms of Common Allergic Reactions, Sensitivities, and Intolerances, Including Anaphylaxis, Asthma, Hives and Other Dermatologic Symptoms, Rhinitis, and Sinusitis

Along with Their Usual Triggers Like Animal Fur, Chemicals, Drugs, Dust, Foods, Insects, Latex, Pollen, and Poison Ivy, Oak, and Sumac; Plus Information on Prevention, Identification, and Treatment

Edited by Allan R. Cook. 611 pages. 1997. 0-7808-0036-2. $78.

Allergies Sourcebook, 2nd Edition

Basic Consumer Health Information about Allergic Disorders, Triggers, Reactions, and Related Symptoms, Including Anaphylaxis, Rhinitis, Sinusitis, Asthma, Dermatitis, Conjunctivitis, and Multiple Chemical Sensitivity

Along with Tips on Diagnosis, Prevention, and Treatment, Statistical Data, a Glossary, and a Directory of Sources for Further Help and Information

Edited by Annemarie S. Muth. 598 pages. 2002. 0-7808-0376-0. $78.

Alternative Medicine Sourcebook, First Edition

Basic Consumer Health Information about Alternatives to Conventional Medicine, Including Acupressure, Acupuncture, Aromatherapy, Ayurveda, Bioelectromagnetics, Environmental Medicine, Essence Therapy, Food and Nutrition Therapy, Herbal Therapy, Homeopathy, Imaging, Massage, Naturopathy, Reflexology, Relaxation and Meditation, Sound Therapy, Vitamin and Mineral Therapy, and Yoga, and More

Edited by Allan R. Cook. 737 pages. 1999. 0-7808-0200-4. $78.

"Recommended reference source."
   —Booklist, American Library Association, Feb '00

"A great addition to the reference collection of every type of library." —American Reference Books Annual, 2000

Alternative Medicine Sourcebook, Second Edition

Basic Consumer Health Information about Alternative and Complementary Medical Practices, Including Acupuncture, Chiropractic, Herbal Medicine, Homeopathy, Naturopathic Medicine, Mind-Body Interventions, Ayurveda, and Other Non-Western Medical Traditions

Along with Facts about such Specific Therapies as Massage Therapy, Aromatherapy, Qigong, Hypnosis, Prayer, Dance, and Art Therapies, a Glossary, and Resources for Further Information

Edited by Dawn D. Matthews. 650 pages. 2002. 0-7808-0605-0. $78.

Alzheimer's, Stroke & 29 Other Neurological Disorders Sourcebook, 1st Edition

Basic Information for the Layperson on 31 Diseases or Disorders Affecting the Brain and Nervous System, First Describing the Illness, Then Listing Symptoms, Diagnostic Methods, and Treatment Options, and Including Statistics on Incidences and Causes

Edited by Frank E. Bair. 579 pages. 1993. 1-55888-748-2. $78.

"Nontechnical reference book that provides reader-friendly information."
   —Family Caregiver Alliance Update, Winter '96

"Should be included in any library's patient education section." —American Reference Books Annual, 1994

"Written in an approachable and accessible style. Recommended for patient education and consumer health collections in health science center and public libraries." —Academic Library Book Review, Dec '93

"It is very handy to have information on more than thirty neurological disorders under one cover, and there is no recent source like it." —Reference Quarterly, American Library Association, Fall '93

SEE ALSO Brain Disorders Sourcebook

Alzheimer's Disease Sourcebook, 2nd Edition

Basic Consumer Health Information about Alzheimer's Disease, Related Disorders, and Other Dementias, Including Multi-Infarct Dementia, AIDS-Related Dementia, Alcoholic Dementia, Huntington's Disease, Delirium, and Confusional States

Along with Reports Detailing Current Research Efforts in Prevention and Treatment, Long-Term Care Issues, and Listings of Sources for Additional Help and Information

Edited by Karen Bellenir. 524 pages. 1999. 0-7808-0223-3. $78.

"Provides a wealth of useful information not otherwise available in one place. This resource is recommended for all types of libraries."
   —American Reference Books Annual, 2000

"Recommended reference source."
   —Booklist, American Library Association, Oct '99

Arthritis Sourcebook

Basic Consumer Health Information about Specific Forms of Arthritis and Related Disorders, Including Rheumatoid Arthritis, Osteoarthritis, Gout, Polymyalgia Rheumatica, Psoriatic Arthritis, Spondyloarthropathies, Juvenile Rheumatoid Arthritis, and Juvenile Ankylosing Spondylitis

Along with Information about Medical, Surgical, and Alternative Treatment Options, and Including Strategies for Coping with Pain, Fatigue, and Stress

Edited by Allan R. Cook. 550 pages. 1998. 0-7808-0201-2. $78.

". . . accessible to the layperson."
—Reference and Research Book News, Feb '99

■

Asthma Sourcebook

Basic Consumer Health Information about Asthma, Including Symptoms, Traditional and Nontraditional Remedies, Treatment Advances, Quality-of-Life Aids, Medical Research Updates, and the Role of Allergies, Exercise, Age, the Environment, and Genetics in the Development of Asthma

Along with Statistical Data, a Glossary, and Directories of Support Groups, and Other Resources for Further Information

Edited by Annemarie S. Muth. 628 pages. 2000. 0-7808-0381-7. $78.

"A worthwhile reference acquisition for public libraries and academic medical libraries whose readers desire a quick introduction to the wide range of asthma information." *— Choice, Association of College & esearch Libraries, Jun '01*

"Recommended reference source."
— Booklist, American Library Association, Feb '01

"Highly recommended." *— The Bookwatch, Jan '01*

"There is much good information for patients and their families who deal with asthma daily."
— American Medical Writers Association Journal, Winter '01

"This informative text is recommended for consumer health collections in public, secondary school, and community college libraries and the libraries of universities with a large undergraduate population."
— American Reference Books Annual, 2001

■

Back & Neck Disorders Sourcebook

Basic Information about Disorders and Injuries of the Spinal Cord and Vertebrae, Including Facts on Chiropractic Treatment, Surgical Interventions, Paralysis, and Rehabilitation

Along with Advice for Preventing Back Trouble

Edited by Karen Bellenir. 548 pages. 1997. 0-7808-0202-0. $78.

"The strength of this work is its basic, easy-to-read format. Recommended."
— Reference and User Services Quarterly, American Library Association, Winter '97

■

Blood & Circulatory Disorders Sourcebook

Basic Information about Blood and Its Components, Anemias, Leukemias, Bleeding Disorders, and Circulatory Disorders, Including Aplastic Anemia, Thalas-

semia, Sickle-Cell Disease, Hemochromatosis, Hemophilia, Von Willebrand Disease, and Vascular Diseases

Along with a Special Section on Blood Transfusions and Blood Supply Safety, a Glossary, and Source Listings for Further Help and Information

Edited by Karen Bellenir and Linda M. Shin. 554 pages. 1998. 0-7808-0203-9. $78.

"Recommended reference source."
— Booklist, American Library Association, Feb '99

"An important reference sourcebook written in simple language for everyday, non-technical users. "
— Reviewer's Bookwatch, Jan '99

■

Brain Disorders Sourcebook

Basic Consumer Health Information about Strokes, Epilepsy, Amyotrophic Lateral Sclerosis (ALS/Lou Gehrig's Disease), Parkinson's Disease, Brain Tumors, Cerebral Palsy, Headache, Tourette Syndrome, and More

Along with Statistical Data, Treatment and Rehabilitation Options, Coping Strategies, Reports on Current Research Initiatives, a Glossary, and Resource Listings for Additional Help and Information

Edited by Karen Bellenir. 481 pages. 1999. 0-7808-0229-2. $78.

"Belongs on the shelves of any library with a consumer health collection." *— E-Streams, Mar '00*

"Recommended reference source."
— Booklist, American Library Association, Oct '99

SEE ALSO *Alzheimer's, Stroke & 29 Other Neurological Disorders Sourcebook, 1st Edition*

■

Breast Cancer Sourcebook

Basic Consumer Health Information about Breast Cancer, Including Diagnostic Methods, Treatment Options, Alternative Therapies, Self-Help Information, Related Health Concerns, Statistical and Demographic Data, and Facts for Men with Breast Cancer

Along with Reports on Current Research Initiatives, a Glossary of Related Medical Terms, and a Directory of Sources for Further Help and Information

Edited by Edward J. Prucha and Karen Bellenir. 580 pages. 2001. 0-7808-0244-6. $78.

"Recommended reference source."
— Booklist, American Library Association, Jan '02

"This reference source is highly recommended. It is quite informative, comprehensive and detailed in nature, and yet it offers practical advice in easy-to-read language. It could be thought of as the 'bible' of breast cancer for the consumer." *— E-Streams, Jan '02*

"From the pros and cons of different screening methods and results to treatment options, *Breast Cancer Sourcebook* provides the latest information on the subject."
— Library Bookwatch, Dec '01

"This thoroughgoing, very readable reference covers all aspects of breast health and cancer.... Readers will find much to consider here. Recommended for all public and patient health collections."

— *Library Journal, Sep '01*

SEE ALSO *Cancer Sourcebook for Women, 1st and 2nd Editions, Women's Health Concerns Sourcebook*

∎

Breastfeeding Sourcebook

Basic Consumer Health Information about the Benefits of Breastmilk, Preparing to Breastfeed, Breastfeeding as a Baby Grows, Nutrition, and More, Including Information on Special Situations and Concerns Such as Mastitis, Illness, Medications, Allergies, Multiple Births, Prematurity, Special Needs, and Adoption

Along with a Glossary and Resources for Additional Help and Information

Edited by Jenni Lynn Colson. 388 pages. 2002. 0-7808-0332-9. $78.

SEE ALSO *Pregnancy & Birth Sourcebook*

∎

Burns Sourcebook

Basic Consumer Health Information about Various Types of Burns and Scalds, Including Flame, Heat, Cold, Electrical, Chemical, and Sun Burns

Along with Information on Short-Term and Long-Term Treatments, Tissue Reconstruction, Plastic Surgery, Prevention Suggestions, and First Aid

Edited by Allan R. Cook. 604 pages. 1999. 0-7808-0204-7. $78.

"This is an exceptional addition to the series and is highly recommended for all consumer health collections, hospital libraries, and academic medical centers."

— *E-Streams, Mar '00*

"This key reference guide is an invaluable addition to all health care and public libraries in confronting this ongoing health issue."

— *American Reference Books Annual, 2000*

"Recommended reference source."

— *Booklist, American Library Association, Dec '99*

SEE ALSO *Skin Disorders Sourcebook*

∎

Cancer Sourcebook, 1st Edition

Basic Information on Cancer Types, Symptoms, Diagnostic Methods, and Treatments, Including Statistics on Cancer Occurrences Worldwide and the Risks Associated with Known Carcinogens and Activities

Edited by Frank E. Bair. 932 pages. 1990. 1-55888-888-8. $78.

Cited in *Reference Sources for Small and Medium-Sized Libraries, American Library Association, 1999*

"Written in nontechnical language. Useful for patients, their families, medical professionals, and librarians."

— *Guide to Reference Books, 1996*

"Designed with the non-medical professional in mind. Libraries and medical facilities interested in patient education should certainly consider adding the *Cancer Sourcebook* to their holdings. This compact collection of reliable information . . . is an invaluable tool for helping patients and patients' families and friends to take the first steps in coping with the many difficulties of cancer."

— *Medical Reference Services Quarterly, Winter '91*

"Specifically created for the nontechnical reader . . . an important resource for the general reader trying to understand the complexities of cancer."

— *American Reference Books Annual, 1991*

"This publication's nontechnical nature and very comprehensive format make it useful for both the general public and undergraduate students."

— *Choice, Association of College and Research Libraries, Oct '90*

∎

New Cancer Sourcebook, 2nd Edition

Basic Information about Major Forms and Stages of Cancer, Featuring Facts about Primary and Secondary Tumors of the Respiratory, Nervous, Lymphatic, Circulatory, Skeletal, and Gastrointestinal Systems, and Specific Organs; Statistical and Demographic Data; Treatment Options; and Strategies for Coping

Edited by Allan R. Cook. 1,313 pages. 1996. 0-7808-0041-9. $78.

"An excellent resource for patients with newly diagnosed cancer and their families. The dialogue is simple, direct, and comprehensive. Highly recommended for patients and families to aid in their understanding of cancer and its treatment."

— *Booklist Health Sciences Supplement, American Library Association, Oct '97*

"The amount of factual and useful information is extensive. The writing is very clear, geared to general readers. Recommended for all levels."

— *Choice, Association of College and Research Libraries, Jan '97*

∎

Cancer Sourcebook, 3rd Edition

Basic Consumer Health Information about Major Forms and Stages of Cancer, Featuring Facts about Primary and Secondary Tumors of the Respiratory, Nervous, Lymphatic, Circulatory, Skeletal, and Gastrointestinal Systems, and Specific Organs

Along with Statistical and Demographic Data, Treatment Options, Strategies for Coping, a Glossary, and a Directory of Sources for Additional Help and Information

Edited by Edward J. Prucha. 1,069 pages. 2000. 0-7808-0227-6. $78.

"This title is recommended for health sciences and public libraries with consumer health collections."

— *E-Streams, Feb '01*

"... can be effectively used by cancer patients and their families who are looking for answers in a language they can understand. Public and hospital libraries should have it on their shelves."
— *American Reference Books Annual, 2001*

"Recommended reference source."
—*Booklist, American Library Association, Dec '00*

■

Cancer Sourcebook for Women, 1st Edition

Basic Information about Specific Forms of Cancer That Affect Women, Featuring Facts about Breast Cancer, Cervical Cancer, Ovarian Cancer, Cancer of the Uterus and Uterine Sarcoma, Cancer of the Vagina, and Cancer of the Vulva; Statistical and Demographic Data; Treatments, Self-Help Management Suggestions, and Current Research Initiatives

Edited by Allan R. Cook and Peter D. Dresser. 524 pages. 1996. 0-7808-0076-1. $78.

"... written in easily understandable, non-technical language. Recommended for public libraries or hospital and academic libraries that collect patient education or consumer health materials."
— *Medical Reference Services Quarterly, Spring '97*

"Would be of value in a consumer health library. . . . written with the health care consumer in mind. Medical jargon is at a minimum, and medical terms are explained in clear, understandable sentences."
— *Bulletin of the Medical Library Association, Oct '96*

"The availability under one cover of all these pertinent publications, grouped under cohesive headings, makes this certainly a most useful sourcebook."
— *Choice, Association of College and Research Libraries, Jun '96*

"Presents a comprehensive knowledge base for general readers. Men and women both benefit from the gold mine of information nestled between the two covers of this book. Recommended."
—*Academic Library Book Review, Summer '96*

"This timely book is highly recommended for consumer health and patient education collections in all libraries."
— *Library Journal, Apr '96*

SEE ALSO Breast Cancer Sourcebook, Women's Health Concerns Sourcebook

■

Cancer Sourcebook for Women, 2nd Edition

Basic Consumer Health Information about Gynecologic Cancers and Related Concerns, Including Cervical Cancer, Endometrial Cancer, Gestational Trophoblastic Tumor, Ovarian Cancer, Uterine Cancer, Vaginal Cancer, Vulvar Cancer, Breast Cancer, and Common Non-Cancerous Uterine Conditions, with Facts about Cancer Risk Factors, Screening and Prevention, Treatment Options, and Reports on Current Research Initiatives

Along with a Glossary of Cancer Terms and a Directory of Resources for Additional Help and Information

Edited by Karen Bellenir. 604 pages. 2002. 0-7808-0226-8. $78.

SEE ALSO Breast Cancer Sourcebook, Women's Health Concerns Sourcebook

■

Cardiovascular Diseases & Disorders Sourcebook, 1st Edition

Basic Information about Cardiovascular Diseases and Disorders, Featuring Facts about the Cardiovascular System, Demographic and Statistical Data, Descriptions of Pharmacological and Surgical Interventions, Lifestyle Modifications, and a Special Section Focusing on Heart Disorders in Children

Edited by Karen Bellenir and Peter D. Dresser. 683 pages. 1995. 0-7808-0032-X. $78.

". . . comprehensive format provides an extensive overview on this subject." — *Choice, Association of College & Research Libraries, Jun '96*

". . . an easily understood, complete, up-to-date resource. This well executed public health tool will make valuable information available to those that need it most, patients and their families. The typeface, sturdy non-reflective paper, and library binding add a feel of quality found wanting in other publications. Highly recommended for academic and general libraries. "
—*Academic Library Book Review, Summer '96*

SEE ALSO Healthy Heart Sourcebook for Women, Heart Diseases & Disorders Sourcebook, 2nd Edition

■

Caregiving Sourcebook

Basic Consumer Health Information for Caregivers, Including a Profile of Caregivers, Caregiving Responsibilities and Concerns, Tips for Specific Conditions, Care Environments, and the Effects of Caregiving

Along with Facts about Legal Issues, Financial Information, and Future Planning, a Glossary, and a Listing of Additional Resources

Edited by Joyce Brennfleck Shannon. 600 pages. 2001. 0-7808-0331-0. $78.

"An ideal addition to the reference collection of any public library. Health sciences information professionals may also want to acquire the *Caregiving Sourcebook* for their hospital or academic library for use as a ready reference tool by health care workers interested in aging and caregiving." —*E-Streams, Jan '02*

"Recommended reference source."
—*Booklist, American Library Association, Oct '01*

Colds, Flu & Other Common Ailments Sourcebook

Basic Consumer Health Information about Common Ailments and Injuries, Including Colds, Coughs, the Flu, Sinus Problems, Headaches, Fever, Nausea and Vomiting, Menstrual Cramps, Diarrhea, Constipation, Hemorrhoids, Back Pain, Dandruff, Dry and Itchy Skin, Cuts, Scrapes, Sprains, Bruises, and More

Along with Information about Prevention, Self-Care, Choosing a Doctor, Over-the-Counter Medications, Folk Remedies, and Alternative Therapies, and Including a Glossary of Important Terms and a Directory of Resources for Further Help and Information

Edited by Chad T. Kimball. 638 pages. 2001. 0-7808-0435-X. $78.

"Will prove valuable to any library seeking to maintain a current, comprehensive reference collection of health resources. . . . Excellent reference."
— The Bookwatch, Aug '01

"Recommended reference source."
— Booklist, American Library Association, July '01

■

Communication Disorders Sourcebook

Basic Information about Deafness and Hearing Loss, Speech and Language Disorders, Voice Disorders, Balance and Vestibular Disorders, and Disorders of Smell, Taste, and Touch

Edited by Linda M. Ross. 533 pages. 1996. 0-7808-0077-X. $78.

"This is skillfully edited and is a welcome resource for the layperson. It should be found in every public and medical library." — Booklist Health Sciences Supplement, American Library Association, Oct '97

■

Congenital Disorders Sourcebook

Basic Information about Disorders Acquired during Gestation, Including Spina Bifida, Hydrocephalus, Cerebral Palsy, Heart Defects, Craniofacial Abnormalities, Fetal Alcohol Syndrome, and More

Along with Current Treatment Options and Statistical Data

Edited by Karen Bellenir. 607 pages. 1997. 0-7808-0205-5. $78.

"Recommended reference source."
— Booklist, American Library Association, Oct '97

SEE ALSO Pregnancy & Birth Sourcebook

■

Consumer Issues in Health Care Sourcebook

Basic Information about Health Care Fundamentals and Related Consumer Issues, Including Exams and Screening Tests, Physician Specialties, Choosing a Doctor, Using Prescription and Over-the-Counter Medica-

tions Safely, Avoiding Health Scams, Managing Common Health Risks in the Home, Care Options for Chronically or Terminally Ill Patients, and a List of Resources for Obtaining Help and Further Information

Edited by Karen Bellenir. 618 pages. 1998. 0-7808-0221-7. $78.

"Both public and academic libraries will want to have a copy in their collection for readers who are interested in self-education on health issues."
— American Reference Books Annual, 2000

"The editor has researched the literature from government agencies and others, saving readers the time and effort of having to do the research themselves. Recommended for public libraries."
— Reference and User Services Quarterly, American Library Association, Spring '99

"Recommended reference source."
— Booklist, American Library Association, Dec '98

■

Contagious & Non-Contagious Infectious Diseases Sourcebook

Basic Information about Contagious Diseases like Measles, Polio, Hepatitis B, and Infectious Mononucleosis, and Non-Contagious Infectious Diseases like Tetanus and Toxic Shock Syndrome, and Diseases Occurring as Secondary Infections Such as Shingles and Reye Syndrome

Along with Vaccination, Prevention, and Treatment Information, and a Section Describing Emerging Infectious Disease Threats

Edited by Karen Bellenir and Peter D. Dresser. 566 pages. 1996. 0-7808-0075-3. $78.

■

Death & Dying Sourcebook

Basic Consumer Health Information for the Layperson about End-of-Life Care and Related Ethical and Legal Issues, Including Chief Causes of Death, Autopsies, Pain Management for the Terminally Ill, Life Support Systems, Insurance, Euthanasia, Assisted Suicide, Hospice Programs, Living Wills, Funeral Planning, Counseling, Mourning, Organ Donation, and Physician Training

Along with Statistical Data, a Glossary, and Listings of Sources for Further Help and Information

Edited by Annemarie S. Muth. 641 pages. 1999. 0-7808-0230-6. $78.

"Public libraries, medical libraries, and academic libraries will all find this sourcebook a useful addition to their collections."
— American Reference Books Annual, 2001

"An extremely useful resource for those concerned with death and dying in the United States."
— Respiratory Care, Nov '00

"Recommended reference source."
— Booklist, American Library Association, Aug '00

"This book is a definite must for all those involved in end-of-life care." — Doody's Review Service, 2000

Diabetes Sourcebook, 1st Edition

Basic Information about Insulin-Dependent and Non-insulin-Dependent Diabetes Mellitus, Gestational Diabetes, and Diabetic Complications, Symptoms, Treatment, and Research Results, Including Statistics on Prevalence, Morbidity, and Mortality

Along with Source Listings for Further Help and Information

Edited by Karen Bellenir and Peter D. Dresser. 827 pages. 1994. 1-55888-751-2. $78.

". . . very informative and understandable for the layperson without being simplistic. It provides a comprehensive overview for laypersons who want a general understanding of the disease or who want to focus on various aspects of the disease."
— Bulletin of the Medical Library Association, Jan '96

Diabetes Sourcebook, 2nd Edition

Basic Consumer Health Information about Type 1 Diabetes (Insulin-Dependent or Juvenile-Onset Diabetes), Type 2 (Noninsulin-Dependent or Adult-Onset Diabetes), Gestational Diabetes, and Related Disorders, Including Diabetes Prevalence Data, Management Issues, the Role of Diet and Exercise in Controlling Diabetes, Insulin and Other Diabetes Medicines, and Complications of Diabetes Such as Eye Diseases, Periodontal Disease, Amputation, and End-Stage Renal Disease

Along with Reports on Current Research Initiatives, a Glossary, and Resource Listings for Further Help and Information

Edited by Karen Bellenir. 688 pages. 1998. 0-7808-0224-1. $78.

"An invaluable reference." *— Library Journal, May '00*

Selected as one of the 250 "Best Health Sciences Books of 1999." *— Doody's Rating Service, Mar-Apr 2000*

"This comprehensive book is an excellent addition for high school, academic, medical, and public libraries. This volume is highly recommended."
—American Reference Books Annual, 2000

"Provides useful information for the general public."
— Healthlines, University of Michigan Health Management Research Center, Sep/Oct '99

". . . provides reliable mainstream medical information . . . belongs on the shelves of any library with a consumer health collection." *— E-Streams, Sep '99*

"Recommended reference source."
— Booklist, American Library Association, Feb '99

Diet & Nutrition Sourcebook, 1st Edition

Basic Information about Nutrition, Including the Dietary Guidelines for Americans, the Food Guide Pyramid, and Their Applications in Daily Diet, Nutritional Advice for Specific Age Groups, Current Nutritional Issues and Controversies, the New Food Label and How to Use It to Promote Healthy Eating, and Recent Developments in Nutritional Research

Edited by Dan R. Harris. 662 pages. 1996. 0-7808-0084-2. $78.

"Useful reference as a food and nutrition sourcebook for the general consumer." *— Booklist Health Sciences Supplement, American Library Association, Oct '97*

"Recommended for public libraries and medical libraries that receive general information requests on nutrition. It is readable and will appeal to those interested in learning more about healthy dietary practices."
— Medical Reference Services Quarterly, Fall '97

"An abundance of medical and social statistics is translated into readable information geared toward the general reader." *— Bookwatch, Mar '97*

"With dozens of questionable diet books on the market, it is so refreshing to find a reliable and factual reference book. Recommended to aspiring professionals, librarians, and others seeking and giving reliable dietary advice. An excellent compilation." *— Choice, Association of College and Research Libraries, Feb '97*

SEE ALSO *Digestive Diseases & Disorders Sourcebook, Gastrointestinal Diseases & Disorders Sourcebook*

Diet & Nutrition Sourcebook, 2nd Edition

Basic Consumer Health Information about Dietary Guidelines, Recommended Daily Intake Values, Vitamins, Minerals, Fiber, Fat, Weight Control, Dietary Supplements, and Food Additives

Along with Special Sections on Nutrition Needs throughout Life and Nutrition for People with Such Specific Medical Concerns as Allergies, High Blood Cholesterol, Hypertension, Diabetes, Celiac Disease, Seizure Disorders, Phenylketonuria (PKU), Cancer, and Eating Disorders, and Including Reports on Current Nutrition Research and Source Listings for Additional Help and Information

Edited by Karen Bellenir. 650 pages. 1999. 0-7808-0228-4. $78.

"This book is an excellent source of basic diet and nutrition information." *— Booklist Health Sciences Supplement, American Library Association, Dec '00*

"This reference document should be in any public library, but it would be a very good guide for beginning students in the health sciences. If the other books in this publisher's series are as good as this, they should all be in the health sciences collections."
—American Reference Books Annual, 2000

"This book is an excellent general nutrition reference for consumers who desire to take an active role in their health care for prevention. Consumers of all ages who select this book can feel confident they are receiving current and accurate information." *— Journal of Nutrition for the Elderly, Vol. 19, No. 4, '00*

"Recommended reference source."
—Booklist, American Library Association, Dec '99

SEE ALSO *Digestive Diseases & Disorders Sourcebook, Gastrointestinal Diseases & Disorders Sourcebook*

Digestive Diseases & Disorders Sourcebook

Basic Consumer Health Information about Diseases and Disorders that Impact the Upper and Lower Digestive System, Including Celiac Disease, Constipation, Crohn's Disease, Cyclic Vomiting Syndrome, Diarrhea, Diverticulosis and Diverticulitis, Gallstones, Heartburn, Hemorrhoids, Hernias, Indigestion (Dyspepsia), Irritable Bowel Syndrome, Lactose Intolerance, Ulcers, and More

Along with Information about Medications and Other Treatments, Tips for Maintaining a Healthy Digestive Tract, a Glossary, and Directory of Digestive Diseases Organizations

Edited by Karen Bellenir. 335 pages. 2000. 0-7808-0327-2. $78.

"This title would be an excellent addition to all public or patient-research libraries."
—*American Reference Books Annual, 2001*

"This title is recommended for public, hospital, and health sciences libraries with consumer health collections."
—*E-Streams, Jul-Aug '00*

"Recommended reference source."
—*Booklist, American Library Association, May '00*

SEE ALSO *Diet & Nutrition Sourcebook, 1st and 2nd Editions, Gastrointestinal Diseases & Disorders Sourcebook*

Disabilities Sourcebook

Basic Consumer Health Information about Physical and Psychiatric Disabilities, Including Descriptions of Major Causes of Disability, Assistive and Adaptive Aids, Workplace Issues, and Accessibility Concerns

Along with Information about the Americans with Disabilities Act, a Glossary, and Resources for Additional Help and Information

Edited by Dawn D. Matthews. 616 pages. 2000. 0-7808-0389-2. $78.

"A much needed addition to the Omnigraphics *Health Reference Series*. A current reference work to provide people with disabilities, their families, caregivers or those who work with them, a broad range of information in one volume, has not been available until now. . . . It is recommended for all public and academic library reference collections."
—*E-Streams, May '01*

"An excellent source book in easy-to-read format covering many current topics; highly recommended for all libraries."
—*Choice, Association of College and Research Libraries, Jan '01*

"Recommended reference source."
—*Booklist, American Library Association, Jul '00*

"An involving, invaluable handbook."
—*The Bookwatch, May '00*

Domestic Violence & Child Abuse Sourcebook

Basic Consumer Health Information about Spousal/Partner, Child, Sibling, Parent, and Elder Abuse, Covering Physical, Emotional, and Sexual Abuse, Teen Dating Violence, and Stalking; Includes Information about Hotlines, Safe Houses, Safety Plans, and Other Resources for Support and Assistance, Community Initiatives, and Reports on Current Directions in Research and Treatment

Along with a Glossary, Sources for Further Reading, and Governmental and Non-Governmental Organizations Contact Information

Edited by Helene Henderson. 1,064 pages. 2001. 0-7808-0235-7. $78.

"This is important information. The Web has many resources but this sourcebook fills an important societal need. I am not aware of any other resources of this type."
—*Doody's Review Service, Sep '01*

"Recommended for all libraries, scholars, and practitioners."
—*Choice, Association of College & Research Libraries, Jul '01*

"Recommended reference source."
—*Booklist, American Library Association, Apr '01*

"Important pick for college-level health reference libraries."
—*The Bookwatch, Mar '01*

"Because this problem is so widespread and because this book includes a lot of issues within one volume, this work is recommended for all public libraries."
—*American Reference Books Annual, 2001*

Drug Abuse Sourcebook

Basic Consumer Health Information about Illicit Substances of Abuse and the Diversion of Prescription Medications, Including Depressants, Hallucinogens, Inhalants, Marijuana, Narcotics, Stimulants, and Anabolic Steroids

Along with Facts about Related Health Risks, Treatment Issues, and Substance Abuse Prevention Programs, a Glossary of Terms, Statistical Data, and Directories of Hotline Services, Self-Help Groups, and Organizations Able to Provide Further Information

Edited by Karen Bellenir. 629 pages. 2000. 0-7808-0242-X. $78.

"Containing a wealth of information, this book will be useful to the college student just beginning to explore the topic of substance abuse. This resource belongs in libraries that serve a lower-division undergraduate or community college clientele as well as the general public."
—*Choice, Association of College and Research Libraries, Jun '01*

"Recommended reference source."
—*Booklist, American Library Association, Feb '01*

"Highly recommended."
—*The Bookwatch, Jan '01*

"Even though there is a plethora of books on drug abuse, this volume is recommended for school, public, and college libraries."
—*American Reference Books Annual, 2001*

Ear, Nose & Throat Disorders Sourcebook

Basic Information about Disorders of the Ears, Nose, Sinus Cavities, Pharynx, and Larynx, Including Ear Infections, Tinnitus, Vestibular Disorders, Allergic and Non-Allergic Rhinitis, Sore Throats, Tonsillitis, and Cancers That Affect the Ears, Nose, Sinuses, and Throat

Along with Reports on Current Research Initiatives, a Glossary of Related Medical Terms, and a Directory of Sources for Further Help and Information

Edited by Karen Bellenir and Linda M. Shin. 576 pages. 1998. 0-7808-0206-3. $78.

"Overall, this sourcebook is helpful for the consumer seeking information on ENT issues. It is recommended for public libraries."
—American Reference Books Annual, 1999

"Recommended reference source."
—Booklist, American Library Association, Dec '98

■

Eating Disorders Sourcebook

Basic Consumer Health Information about Eating Disorders, Including Information about Anorexia Nervosa, Bulimia Nervosa, Binge Eating, Body Dysmorphic Disorder, Pica, Laxative Abuse, and Night Eating Syndrome

Along with Information about Causes, Adverse Effects, and Treatment and Prevention Issues, and Featuring a Section on Concerns Specific to Children and Adolescents, a Glossary, and Resources for Further Help and Information

Edited by Dawn D. Matthews. 322 pages. 2001. 0-7808-0335-3. $78.

"This volume is another convenient collection of excerpted articles. Recommended for school and public library patrons; lower-division undergraduates; and two-year technical program students."
—Choice, Association of College & Research Libraries, Jan '02

"Recommended reference source." *—Booklist, American Library Association, Oct '01*

■

Endocrine & Metabolic Disorders Sourcebook

Basic Information for the Layperson about Pancreatic and Insulin-Related Disorders Such as Pancreatitis, Diabetes, and Hypoglycemia; Adrenal Gland Disorders Such as Cushing's Syndrome, Addison's Disease, and Congenital Adrenal Hyperplasia; Pituitary Gland Disorders Such as Growth Hormone Deficiency, Acromegaly, and Pituitary Tumors; Thyroid Disorders Such as Hypothyroidism, Graves' Disease, Hashimoto's Disease, and Goiter; Hyperparathyroidism; and Other Diseases and Syndromes of Hormone Imbalance or Metabolic Dysfunction

Along with Reports on Current Research Initiatives

Edited by Linda M. Shin. 574 pages. 1998. 0-7808-0207-1. $78.

"Omnigraphics has produced another needed resource for health information consumers."
—American Reference Books Annual, 2000

"Recommended reference source."
—Booklist, American Library Association, Dec '98

■

Environmentally Induced Disorders Sourcebook

Basic Information about Diseases and Syndromes Linked to Exposure to Pollutants and Other Substances in Outdoor and Indoor Environments Such as Lead, Asbestos, Formaldehyde, Mercury, Emissions, Noise, and More

Edited by Allan R. Cook. 620 pages. 1997. 0-7808-0083-4. $78.

"Recommended reference source."
—Booklist, American Library Association, Sep '98

"This book will be a useful addition to anyone's library." *—Choice Health Sciences Supplement, Association of College and Research Libraries, May '98*

". . . a good survey of numerous environmentally induced physical disorders . . . a useful addition to anyone's library."
—Doody's Health Sciences Book Reviews, Jan '98

". . . provide[s] introductory information from the best authorities around. Since this volume covers topics that potentially affect everyone, it will surely be one of the most frequently consulted volumes in the *Health Reference Series*." *—Rettig on Reference, Nov '97*

■

Ethnic Diseases Sourcebook

Basic Consumer Health Information for Ethnic and Racial Minority Groups in the United States, Including General Health Indicators and Behaviors, Ethnic Diseases, Genetic Testing, the Impact of Chronic Diseases, Women's Health, Mental Health Issues, and Preventive Health Care Services

Along with a Glossary and a Listing of Additional Resources

Edited by Joyce Brennfleck Shannon. 664 pages. 2001. 0-7808-0336-1. $78.

"Recommended for health sciences libraries where public health programs are a priority."
—E-Streams, Jan '02

"Recommended reference source."
—Booklist, American Library Association, Oct '01

"Will prove valuable to any library seeking to maintain a current, comprehensive reference collection of health resources. . . . An excellent source of health information about genetic disorders which affect particular ethnic and racial minorities in the U.S."
—The Bookwatch, Aug '01

Family Planning Sourcebook

Basic Consumer Health Information about Planning for Pregnancy and Contraception, Including Traditional Methods, Barrier Methods, Hormonal Methods, Permanent Methods, Future Methods, Emergency Contraception, and Birth Control Choices for Women at Each Stage of Life

Along with Statistics, a Glossary, and Sources of Additional Information

Edited by Amy Marcaccio Keyzer. 520 pages. 2001. 0-7808-0379-5. $78.

"Recommended reference source."
— Booklist, American Library Association, Oct '01

"Will prove valuable to any library seeking to maintain a current, comprehensive reference collection of health resources. . . . Excellent reference."
— The Bookwatch, Aug '01

SEE ALSO Pregnancy & Birth Sourcebook

■

Fitness & Exercise Sourcebook, 1st Edition

Basic Information on Fitness and Exercise, Including Fitness Activities for Specific Age Groups, Exercise for People with Specific Medical Conditions, How to Begin a Fitness Program in Running, Walking, Swimming, Cycling, and Other Athletic Activities, and Recent Research in Fitness and Exercise

Edited by Dan R. Harris. 663 pages. 1996. 0-7808-0186-5. $78.

"A good resource for general readers."   — Choice, Association of College and Research Libraries, Nov '97

"The perennial popularity of the topic . . . make this an appealing selection for public libraries."
— Rettig on Reference, Jun/Jul '97

■

Fitness & Exercise Sourcebook, 2nd Edition

Basic Consumer Health Information about the Fundamentals of Fitness and Exercise, Including How to Begin and Maintain a Fitness Program, Fitness as a Lifestyle, the Link between Fitness and Diet, Advice for Specific Groups of People, Exercise as It Relates to Specific Medical Conditions, and Recent Research in Fitness and Exercise

Along with a Glossary of Important Terms and Resources for Additional Help and Information

Edited by Kristen M. Gledhill. 646 pages. 2001. 0-7808-0334-5. $78.

"Highly recommended for public, consumer, and school grades fourth through college."
— E-Streams, Nov '01

"Recommended reference source."   — Booklist, American Library Association, Oct '01

"The information appears quite comprehensive and is considered reliable. . . . This second edition is a welcomed addition to the series."
— Doody's Review Service, Sep '01

"This reference is a valuable choice for those who desire a broad source of information on exercise, fitness, and chronic-disease prevention through a healthy lifestyle."   — American Medical Writers Association Journal, Fall '01

"Will prove valuable to any library seeking to maintain a current, comprehensive reference collection of health resources. . . . Excellent reference."
— The Bookwatch, Aug '01

■

Food & Animal Borne Diseases Sourcebook

Basic Information about Diseases That Can Be Spread to Humans through the Ingestion of Contaminated Food or Water or by Contact with Infected Animals and Insects, Such as Botulism, E. Coli, Hepatitis A, Trichinosis, Lyme Disease, and Rabies

Along with Information Regarding Prevention and Treatment Methods, and Including a Special Section for International Travelers Describing Diseases Such as Cholera, Malaria, Travelers' Diarrhea, and Yellow Fever, and Offering Recommendations for Avoiding Illness

Edited by Karen Bellenir and Peter D. Dresser. 535 pages. 1995. 0-7808-0033-8. $78.

"Targeting general readers and providing them with a single, comprehensive source of information on selected topics, this book continues, with the excellent caliber of its predecessors, to catalog topical information on health matters of general interest. Readable and thorough, this valuable resource is highly recommended for all libraries."
— Academic Library Book Review, Summer '96

"A comprehensive collection of authoritative information."   — Emergency Medical Services, Oct '95

■

Food Safety Sourcebook

Basic Consumer Health Information about the Safe Handling of Meat, Poultry, Seafood, Eggs, Fruit Juices, and Other Food Items, and Facts about Pesticides, Drinking Water, Food Safety Overseas, and the Onset, Duration, and Symptoms of Foodborne Illnesses, Including Types of Pathogenic Bacteria, Parasitic Protozoa, Worms, Viruses, and Natural Toxins

Along with the Role of the Consumer, the Food Handler, and the Government in Food Safety; a Glossary, and Resources for Additional Help and Information

Edited by Dawn D. Matthews. 339 pages. 1999. 0-7808-0326-4. $78.

"This book is recommended for public libraries and universities with home economic and food science programs."   — E-Streams, Nov '00

"Recommended reference source."
— Booklist, American Library Association, May '00

"This book takes the complex issues of food safety and foodborne pathogens and presents them in an easily understood manner. [It does] an excellent job of covering a large and often confusing topic."
—*American Reference Books Annual, 2000*

■

Forensic Medicine Sourcebook

Basic Consumer Information for the Layperson about Forensic Medicine, Including Crime Scene Investigation, Evidence Collection and Analysis, Expert Testimony, Computer-Aided Criminal Identification, Digital Imaging in the Courtroom, DNA Profiling, Accident Reconstruction, Autopsies, Ballistics, Drugs and Explosives Detection, Latent Fingerprints, Product Tampering, and Questioned Document Examination

Along with Statistical Data, a Glossary of Forensics Terminology, and Listings of Sources for Further Help and Information

Edited by Annemarie S. Muth. 574 pages. 1999. 0-7808-0232-2. $78.

"Given the expected widespread interest in its content and its easy to read style, this book is recommended for most public and all college and university libraries."
— *E-Streams, Feb '01*

"Recommended for public libraries."
—*Reference & User Services Quarterly, American Library Association, Spring 2000*

"Recommended reference source."
—*Booklist, American Library Association, Feb '00*

"A wealth of information, useful statistics, references are up-to-date and extremely complete. This wonderful collection of data will help students who are interested in a career in any type of forensic field. It is a great resource for attorneys who need information about types of expert witnesses needed in a particular case. It also offers useful information for fiction and nonfiction writers whose work involves a crime. A fascinating compilation. All levels." — *Choice, Association of College and Research Libraries, Jan 2000*

"There are several items that make this book attractive to consumers who are seeking certain forensic data. . . . This is a useful current source for those seeking general forensic medical answers."
—*American Reference Books Annual, 2000*

■

Gastrointestinal Diseases & Disorders Sourcebook

Basic Information about Gastroesophageal Reflux Disease (Heartburn), Ulcers, Diverticulosis, Irritable Bowel Syndrome, Crohn's Disease, Ulcerative Colitis, Diarrhea, Constipation, Lactose Intolerance, Hemorrhoids, Hepatitis, Cirrhosis, and Other Digestive Problems, Featuring Statistics, Descriptions of Symptoms, and Current Treatment Methods of Interest for Persons Living with Upper and Lower Gastrointestinal Maladies

Edited by Linda M. Ross. 413 pages. 1996. 0-7808-0078-8. $78.

". . . very readable form. The successful editorial work that brought this material together into a useful and understandable reference makes accessible to all readers information that can help them more effectively understand and obtain help for digestive tract problems."
— *Choice, Association of College and Research Libraries, Feb '97*

SEE ALSO *Diet & Nutrition Sourcebook, 1st and 2nd Editions, Digestive Diseases & Disorders*

■

Genetic Disorders Sourcebook, 1st Edition

Basic Information about Heritable Diseases and Disorders Such as Down Syndrome, PKU, Hemophilia, Von Willebrand Disease, Gaucher Disease, Tay-Sachs Disease, and Sickle-Cell Disease, Along with Information about Genetic Screening, Gene Therapy, Home Care, and Including Source Listings for Further Help and Information on More Than 300 Disorders

Edited by Karen Bellenir. 642 pages. 1996. 0-7808-0034-6. $78.

"Recommended for undergraduate libraries or libraries that serve the public."
— *Science & Technology Libraries, Vol. 18, No. 1, '99*

"Provides essential medical information to both the general public and those diagnosed with a serious or fatal genetic disease or disorder." —*Choice, Association of College and Research Libraries, Jan '97*

"Geared toward the lay public. It would be well placed in all public libraries and in those hospital and medical libraries in which access to genetic references is limited." —*Doody's Health Sciences Book Review, Oct '96*

■

Genetic Disorders Sourcebook, 2nd Edition

Basic Consumer Health Information about Hereditary Diseases and Disorders, Including Cystic Fibrosis, Down Syndrome, Hemophilia, Huntington's Disease, Sickle Cell Anemia, and More; Facts about Genes, Gene Research and Therapy, Genetic Screening, Ethics of Gene Testing, Genetic Counseling, and Advice on Coping and Caring

Along with a Glossary of Genetic Terminology and a Resource List for Help, Support, and Further Information

Edited by Kathy Massimini. 768 pages. 2001. 0-7808-0241-1. $78.

"Recommended for public libraries and medical and hospital libraries with consumer health collections."
—*E-Streams, May '01*

"Recommended reference source."
— *Booklist, American Library Association, Apr '01*

"Important pick for college-level health reference libraries." —*The Bookwatch, Mar '01*

Head Trauma Sourcebook

Basic Information for the Layperson about Open-Head and Closed-Head Injuries, Treatment Advances, Recovery, and Rehabilitation

Along with Reports on Current Research Initiatives

Edited by Karen Bellenir. 414 pages. 1997. 0-7808-0208-X. $78.

Headache Sourcebook

Basic Consumer Health Information about Migraine, Tension, Cluster, Rebound and Other Types of Headaches, with Facts about the Cause and Prevention of Headaches, the Effects of Stress and the Environment, Headaches during Pregnancy and Menopause, and Childhood Headaches

Along with a Glossary and Other Resources for Additional Help and Information

Edited by Dawn D. Matthews. 362 pages. 2002. 0-7808-0337-X. $78.

Health Insurance Sourcebook

Basic Information about Managed Care Organizations, Traditional Fee-for-Service Insurance, Insurance Portability and Pre-Existing Conditions Clauses, Medicare, Medicaid, Social Security, and Military Health Care

Along with Information about Insurance Fraud

Edited by Wendy Wilcox. 530 pages. 1997. 0-7808-0222-5. $78.

"Particularly useful because it brings much of this information together in one volume. This book will be a handy reference source in the health sciences library, hospital library, college and university library, and medium to large public library."
— *Medical Reference Services Quarterly, Fall '98*

Awarded "Books of the Year Award"
— *American Journal of Nursing, 1997*

"The layout of the book is particularly helpful as it provides easy access to reference material. A most useful addition to the vast amount of information about health insurance. The use of data from U.S. government agencies is most commendable. Useful in a library or learning center for healthcare professional students."
— *Doody's Health Sciences Book Reviews, Nov '97*

Health Reference Series Cumulative Index 1999

A Comprehensive Index to the Individual Volumes of the Health Reference Series, Including a Subject Index, Name Index, Organization Index, and Publication Index

Along with a Master List of Acronyms and Abbreviations

Edited by Edward J. Prucha, Anne Holmes, and Robert Rudnick. 990 pages. 2000. 0-7808-0382-5. $78.

"This volume will be most helpful in libraries that have a relatively complete collection of the Health Reference Series." — *American Reference Books Annual, 2001*

"Essential for collections that hold any of the numerous *Health Reference Series* titles."
— *Choice, Association of College and Research Libraries, Nov '00*

Healthy Aging Sourcebook

Basic Consumer Health Information about Maintaining Health through the Aging Process, Including Advice on Nutrition, Exercise, and Sleep, Help in Making Decisions about Midlife Issues and Retirement, and Guidance Concerning Practical and Informed Choices in Health Consumerism

Along with Data Concerning the Theories of Aging, Different Experiences in Aging by Minority Groups, and Facts about Aging Now and Aging in the Future; and Featuring a Glossary, a Guide to Consumer Help, Additional Suggested Reading, and Practical Resource Directory

Edited by Jenifer Swanson. 536 pages. 1999. 0-7808-0390-6. $78.

"Recommended reference source."
— *Booklist, American Library Association, Feb '00*

SEE ALSO *Physical & Mental Issues in Aging Sourcebook*

Healthy Heart Sourcebook for Women

Basic Consumer Health Information about Cardiac Issues Specific to Women, Including Facts about Major Risk Factors and Prevention, Treatment and Control Strategies, and Important Dietary Issues

Along with a Special Section Regarding the Pros and Cons of Hormone Replacement Therapy and Its Impact on Heart Health, and Additional Help, Including Recipes, a Glossary, and a Directory of Resources

Edited by Dawn D. Matthews. 336 pages. 2000. 0-7808-0329-9. $78.

"A good reference source and recommended for all public, academic, medical, and hospital libraries."
— *Medical Reference Services Quarterly, Summer '01*

"Because of the lack of information specific to women on this topic, this book is recommended for public libraries and consumer libraries."
— *American Reference Books Annual, 2001*

"Contains very important information about coronary artery disease that all women should know. The information is current and presented in an easy-to-read format. The book will make a good addition to any library." — *American Medical Writers Association Journal, Summer '00*

"Important, basic reference."
— *Reviewer's Bookwatch, Jul '00*

SEE ALSO *Cardiovascular Diseases & Disorders Sourcebook, 1st Edition, Heart Diseases & Disorders*

■

Heart Diseases & Disorders Sourcebook, 2nd Edition

Basic Consumer Health Information about Heart Attacks, Angina, Rhythm Disorders, Heart Failure, Valve Disease, Congenital Heart Disorders, and More, Including Descriptions of Surgical Procedures and Other Interventions, Medications, Cardiac Rehabilitation, Risk Identification, and Prevention Tips

Along with Statistical Data, Reports on Current Research Initiatives, a Glossary of Cardiovascular Terms, and Resource Directory

Edited by Karen Bellenir. 612 pages. 2000. 0-7808-0238-1. $78.

"This work stands out as an imminently accessible resource for the general public. It is recommended for the reference and circulating shelves of school, public, and academic libraries."
— *American Reference Books Annual, 2001*

"Recommended reference source."
— *Booklist, American Library Association, Dec '00*

"Provides comprehensive coverage of matters related to the heart. This title is recommended for health sciences and public libraries with consumer health collections."
— *E-Streams, Oct '00*

SEE ALSO *Cardiovascular Diseases & Disorders Sourcebook, 1st Edition; Healthy Heart Sourcebook for Women*

■

Household Safety Sourcebook

Basic Consumer Health Information about Household Safety, Including Information about Poisons, Chemicals, Fire, and Water Hazards in the Home

Along with Advice about the Safe Use of Home Maintenance Equipment, Choosing Toys and Nursery Furniture, Holiday and Recreation Safety, a Glossary, and Resources for Further Help and Information

Edited by Dawn D. Matthews. 606 pages. 2002. 0-7808-0338-8. $78.

■

Immune System Disorders Sourcebook

Basic Information about Lupus, Multiple Sclerosis, Guillain-Barré Syndrome, Chronic Granulomatous Disease, and More

Along with Statistical and Demographic Data and Reports on Current Research Initiatives

Edited by Allan R. Cook. 608 pages. 1997. 0-7808-0209-8. $78.

Infant & Toddler Health Sourcebook

Basic Consumer Health Information about the Physical and Mental Development of Newborns, Infants, and Toddlers, Including Neonatal Concerns, Nutrition Recommendations, Immunization Schedules, Common Pediatric Disorders, Assessments and Milestones, Safety Tips, and Advice for Parents and Other Caregivers

Along with a Glossary of Terms and Resource Listings for Additional Help

Edited by Jenifer Swanson. 585 pages. 2000. 0-7808-0246-2. $78.

"As a reference for the general public, this would be useful in any library."   — *E-Streams, May '01*

"Recommended reference source."
— *Booklist, American Library Association, Feb '01*

"This is a good source for general use."
— *American Reference Books Annual, 2001*

■

Injury & Trauma Sourcebook

Basic Consumer Health Information about the Impact of Injury, the Diagnosis and Treatment of Common and Traumatic Injuries, Emergency Care, and Specific Injuries Related to Home, Community, Workplace, Transportation, and Recreation

Along with Guidelines for Injury Prevention, a Glossary, and a Directory of Additional Resources

Edited by Joyce Brennfleck Shannon. 696 pages. 2002. 0-7808-0421-X. $78.

■

Kidney & Urinary Tract Diseases & Disorders Sourcebook

Basic Information about Kidney Stones, Urinary Incontinence, Bladder Disease, End Stage Renal Disease, Dialysis, and More

Along with Statistical and Demographic Data and Reports on Current Research Initiatives

Edited by Linda M. Ross. 602 pages. 1997. 0-7808-0079-6. $78.

■

Learning Disabilities Sourcebook

Basic Information about Disorders Such as Dyslexia, Visual and Auditory Processing Deficits, Attention Deficit/Hyperactivity Disorder, and Autism

Along with Statistical and Demographic Data, Reports on Current Research Initiatives, an Explanation of the Assessment Process, and a Special Section for Adults with Learning Disabilities

Edited by Linda M. Shin. 579 pages. 1998. 0-7808-0210-1. $78.

Named "Outstanding Reference Book of 1999."
— *New York Public Library, Feb 2000*

■

Liver Disorders Sourcebook

Basic Consumer Health Information about the Liver and How It Works; Liver Diseases, Including Cancer, Cirrhosis, Hepatitis, and Toxic and Drug Related Diseases; Tips for Maintaining a Healthy Liver; Laboratory Tests, Radiology Tests, and Facts about Liver Transplantation

Along with a Section on Support Groups, a Glossary, and Resource Listings

Edited by Joyce Brennfleck Shannon. 591 pages. 2000. 0-7808-0383-3. $78.

■

Lung Disorders Sourcebook

Basic Consumer Health Information about Emphysema, Pneumonia, Tuberculosis, Asthma, Cystic Fibrosis, and Other Lung Disorders, Including Facts about Diagnostic Procedures, Treatment Strategies, Disease Prevention Efforts, and Such Risk Factors as Smoking, Air Pollution, and Exposure to Asbestos, Radon, and Other Agents

Along with a Glossary and Resources for Additional Help and Information

Edited by Dawn D. Matthews. 678 pages. 2002. 0-7808-0339-6. $78.

Medical Tests Sourcebook

Basic Consumer Health Information about Medical Tests, Including Periodic Health Exams, General Screening Tests, Tests You Can Do at Home, Findings of the U.S. Preventive Services Task Force, X-ray and Radiology Tests, Electrical Tests, Tests of Blood and Other Body Fluids and Tissues, Scope Tests, Lung Tests, Genetic Tests, Pregnancy Tests, Newborn Screening Tests, Sexually Transmitted Disease Tests, and Computer Aided Diagnoses

Along with a Section on Paying for Medical Tests, a Glossary, and Resource Listings

Edited by Joyce Brennfleck Shannon. 691 pages. 1999. 0-7808-0243-8. $78.

■

Men's Health Concerns Sourcebook

Basic Information about Health Issues That Affect Men, Featuring Facts about the Top Causes of Death in Men, Including Heart Disease, Stroke, Cancers, Prostate Disorders, Chronic Obstructive Pulmonary Disease, Pneumonia and Influenza, Human Immunodeficiency Virus and Acquired Immune Deficiency Syndrome, Diabetes Mellitus, Stress, Suicide, Accidents and Homicides; and Facts about Common Concerns for Men, Including Impotence, Contraception, Circumcision, Sleep Disorders, Snoring, Hair Loss, Diet, Nutrition, Exercise, Kidney and Urological Disorders, and Backaches

Edited by Allan R. Cook. 738 pages. 1998. 0-7808-0212-8. $78.

■

Mental Health Disorders Sourcebook, 1st Edition

Basic Information about Schizophrenia, Depression, Bipolar Disorder, Panic Disorder, Obsessive-Compulsive Disorder, Phobias and Other Anxiety Disorders, Paranoia and Other Personality Disorders, Eating Disorders, and Sleep Disorders

Along with Information about Treatment and Therapies

Edited by Karen Bellenir. 548 pages. 1995. 0-7808-0040-0. $78.

"This is an excellent new book . . . written in easy-to-understand language."
— *Booklist Health Sciences Supplement, American Library Association, Oct '97*

". . . useful for public and academic libraries and consumer health collections."
— *Medical Reference Services Quarterly, Spring '97*

"The great strengths of the book are its readability and its inclusion of places to find more information. Especially recommended."   — *Reference Quarterly, American Library Association, Winter '96*

". . . a good resource for a consumer health library."
—*Bulletin of the Medical Library Association, Oct '96*

"The information is data-based and couched in brief, concise language that avoids jargon. . . . a useful reference source."   — *Readings, Sep '96*

"The text is well organized and adequately written for its target audience."   — *Choice, Association of College and Research Libraries, Jun '96*

". . . provides information on a wide range of mental disorders, presented in nontechnical language."
— *Exceptional Child Education Resources, Spring '96*

"Recommended for public and academic libraries."
— *Reference Book Review, 1996*

■

Mental Health Disorders Sourcebook, 2nd Edition

Basic Consumer Health Information about Anxiety Disorders, Depression and Other Mood Disorders, Eating Disorders, Personality Disorders, Schizophrenia, and More, Including Disease Descriptions, Treatment Options, and Reports on Current Research Initiatives

Along with Statistical Data, Tips for Maintaining Mental Health, a Glossary, and Directory of Sources for Additional Help and Information

Edited by Karen Bellenir. 605 pages. 2000. 0-7808-0240-3. $78.

"Well organized and well written."
—*American Reference Books Annual, 2001*

"Recommended reference source."
—*Booklist, American Library Association, Jun '00*

■

Mental Retardation Sourcebook

Basic Consumer Health Information about Mental Retardation and Its Causes, Including Down Syndrome, Fetal Alcohol Syndrome, Fragile X Syndrome, Genetic Conditions, Injury, and Environmental Sources

Along with Preventive Strategies, Parenting Issues, Educational Implications, Health Care Needs, Employment and Economic Matters, Legal Issues, a Glossary, and a Resource Listing for Additional Help and Information

Edited by Joyce Brennfleck Shannon. 642 pages. 2000. 0-7808-0377-9. $78.

"Public libraries will find the book useful for reference and as a beginning research point for students, parents, and caregivers."
—*American Reference Books Annual, 2001*

"The strength of this work is that it compiles many basic fact sheets and addresses for further information in one volume. It is intended and suitable for the general public. This sourcebook is relevant to any collection providing health information to the general public."
—*E-Streams, Nov '00*

"From preventing retardation to parenting and family challenges, this covers health, social and legal issues and will prove an invaluable overview."
— *Reviewer's Bookwatch, Jul '00*

■

Obesity Sourcebook

Basic Consumer Health Information about Diseases and Other Problems Associated with Obesity, and Including Facts about Risk Factors, Prevention Issues, and Management Approaches

Along with Statistical and Demographic Data, Information about Special Populations, Research Updates, a Glossary, and Source Listings for Further Help and Information

Edited by Wilma Caldwell and Chad T. Kimball. 376 pages. 2001. 0-7808-0333-7. $78.

"This is a very useful resource book for the lay public."
—*Doody's Review Service, Nov '01*

"Well suited for the health reference collection of a public library or an academic health science library that serves the general population."   —*E-Streams, Sep '01*

"Recommended reference source."
—*Booklist, American Library Association, Apr '01*

" Recommended pick both for specialty health library collections and any general consumer health reference collection."   — *The Bookwatch, Apr '01*

■

Ophthalmic Disorders Sourcebook

Basic Information about Glaucoma, Cataracts, Macular Degeneration, Strabismus, Refractive Disorders, and More

Along with Statistical and Demographic Data and Reports on Current Research Initiatives

Edited by Linda M. Ross. 631 pages. 1996. 0-7808-0081-8. $78.

■

Oral Health Sourcebook

Basic Information about Diseases and Conditions Affecting Oral Health, Including Cavities, Gum Disease, Dry Mouth, Oral Cancers, Fever Blisters, Canker Sores, Oral Thrush, Bad Breath, Temporomandibular Disorders, and other Craniofacial Syndromes

Along with Statistical Data on the Oral Health of Americans, Oral Hygiene, Emergency First Aid, In-

formation on Treatment Procedures and Methods of Replacing Lost Teeth

Edited by Allan R. Cook. 558 pages. 1997. 0-7808-0082-6. $78.

"Unique source which will fill a gap in dental sources for patients and the lay public. A valuable reference tool even in a library with thousands of books on dentistry. Comprehensive, clear, inexpensive, and easy to read and use. It fills an enormous gap in the health care literature." *— Reference and User Services Quarterly, American Library Association, Summer '98*

"Recommended reference source."
— Booklist, American Library Association, Dec '97

■

Osteoporosis Sourcebook

Basic Consumer Health Information about Primary and Secondary Osteoporosis and Juvenile Osteoporosis and Related Conditions, Including Fibrous Dysplasia, Gaucher Disease, Hyperthyroidism, Hypophosphatasia, Myeloma, Osteopetrosis, Osteogenesis Imperfecta, and Paget's Disease

Along with Information about Risk Factors, Treatments, Traditional and Non-Traditional Pain Management, a Glossary of Related Terms, and a Directory of Resources

Edited by Allan R. Cook. 584 pages. 2001. 0-7808-0239-X. $78.

"This would be a book to be kept in a staff or patient library. The targeted audience is the layperson, but the therapist who needs a quick bit of information on a particular topic will also find the book useful."
—Physical Therapy, Jan '02

"Recommended for all public libraries and general health collections, especially those supporting patient education or consumer health programs."
—E-Streams, Nov '01

"Will prove valuable to any library seeking to maintain a current, comprehensive reference collection of health resources. . . . From prevention to treatment and associated conditions, this provides an excellent survey."
—The Bookwatch, Aug '01

"Recommended reference source."
—Booklist, American Library Association, July '01

SEE ALSO *Women's Health Concerns Sourcebook*

■

Pain Sourcebook, 1st Edition

Basic Information about Specific Forms of Acute and Chronic Pain, Including Headaches, Back Pain, Muscular Pain, Neuralgia, Surgical Pain, and Cancer Pain

Along with Pain Relief Options Such as Analgesics, Narcotics, Nerve Blocks, Transcutaneous Nerve Stimulation, and Alternative Forms of Pain Control, Including Biofeedback, Imaging, Behavior Modification, and Relaxation Techniques

Edited by Allan R. Cook. 667 pages. 1997. 0-7808-0213-6. $78.

"The text is readable, easily understood, and well indexed. This excellent volume belongs in all patient education libraries, consumer health sections of public libraries, and many personal collections."
—American Reference Books Annual, 1999

"A beneficial reference." *—Booklist Health Sciences Supplement, American Library Association, Oct '98*

"The information is basic in terms of scholarship and is appropriate for general readers. Written in journalistic style . . . intended for non-professionals. Quite thorough in its coverage of different pain conditions and summarizes the latest clinical information regarding pain treatment." *— Choice, Association of College and Research Libraries, Jun '98*

"Recommended reference source."
—Booklist, American Library Association, Mar '98

■

Pain Sourcebook, 2nd Edition

Basic Consumer Health Information about Specific Forms of Acute and Chronic Pain, Including Muscle and Skeletal Pain, Nerve Pain, Cancer Pain, and Disorders Characterized by Pain, Such as Fibromyalgia, Shingles, Angina, Arthritis, and Headaches

Along with Information about Pain Medications and Management Techniques, Complementary and Alternative Pain Relief Options, Tips for People Living with Chronic Pain, a Glossary, and a Directory of Sources for Further Information

Edited by Karen Bellenir. 650 pages. 2002. 0-7808-0612-3. $78.

■

Pediatric Cancer Sourcebook

Basic Consumer Health Information about Leukemias, Brain Tumors, Sarcomas, Lymphomas, and Other Cancers in Infants, Children, and Adolescents, Including Descriptions of Cancers, Treatments, and Coping Strategies

Along with Suggestions for Parents, Caregivers, and Concerned Relatives, a Glossary of Cancer Terms, and Resource Listings

Edited by Edward J. Prucha. 587 pages. 1999. 0-7808-0245-4. $78.

"An excellent source of information. Recommended for public, hospital, and health science libraries with consumer health collections." *— E-Streams, Jun '00*

"Recommended reference source."
—Booklist, American Library Association, Feb '00

"A valuable addition to all libraries specializing in health services and many public libraries."
—American Reference Books Annual, 2000

Physical & Mental Issues in Aging Sourcebook

Basic Consumer Health Information on Physical and Mental Disorders Associated with the Aging Process, Including Concerns about Cardiovascular Disease, Pulmonary Disease, Oral Health, Digestive Disorders, Musculoskeletal and Skin Disorders, Metabolic Changes, Sexual and Reproductive Issues, and Changes in Vision, Hearing, and Other Senses

Along with Data about Longevity and Causes of Death, Information on Acute and Chronic Pain, Descriptions of Mental Concerns, a Glossary of Terms, and Resource Listings for Additional Help

Edited by Jenifer Swanson. 660 pages. 1999. 0-7808-0233-0. $78.

"This is a treasure of health information for the layperson."   — Choice Health Sciences Supplement, Association of College & Research Libraries, May 2000

"Recommended for public libraries."
— American Reference Books Annual, 2000

"Recommended reference source."
— Booklist, American Library Association, Oct '99

SEE ALSO Healthy Aging Sourcebook

■

Podiatry Sourcebook

Basic Consumer Health Information about Foot Conditions, Diseases, and Injuries, Including Bunions, Corns, Calluses, Athlete's Foot, Plantar Warts, Hammertoes and Clawtoes, Clubfoot, Heel Pain, Gout, and More

Along with Facts about Foot Care, Disease Prevention, Foot Safety, Choosing a Foot Care Specialist, a Glossary of Terms, and Resource Listings for Additional Information

Edited by M. Lisa Weatherford. 380 pages. 2001. 0-7808-0215-2. $78.

■

Pregnancy & Birth Sourcebook

Basic Information about Planning for Pregnancy, Maternal Health, Fetal Growth and Development, Labor and Delivery, Postpartum and Perinatal Care, Pregnancy in Mothers with Special Concerns, and Disorders of Pregnancy, Including Genetic Counseling, Nutrition and Exercise, Obstetrical Tests, Pregnancy Discomfort, Multiple Births, Cesarean Sections, Medical Testing of Newborns, Breastfeeding, Gestational Diabetes, and Ectopic Pregnancy

Edited by Heather E. Aldred. 737 pages. 1997. 0-7808-0216-0. $78.

"A well-organized handbook. Recommended."
— Choice, Association of College and Research Libraries, Apr '98

"Recommended reference source."
— Booklist, American Library Association, Mar '98

"Recommended for public libraries."
— American Reference Books Annual, 1998

SEE ALSO Congenital Disorders Sourcebook, Family Planning Sourcebook

■

Prostate Cancer Sourcebook

Basic Consumer Health Information about Prostate Cancer, Including Information about the Associated Risk Factors, Detection, Diagnosis, and Treatment of Prostate Cancer

Along with Information on Non-Malignant Prostate Conditions, and Featuring a Section Listing Support and Treatment Centers and a Glossary of Related Terms

Edited by Dawn D. Matthews. 358 pages. 2001. 0-7808-0324-8. $78.

"Recommended reference source."
— Booklist, American Library Association, Jan '02

Public Health Sourcebook

Basic Information about Government Health Agencies, Including National Health Statistics and Trends, Healthy People 2000 Program Goals and Objectives, the Centers for Disease Control and Prevention, the Food and Drug Administration, and the National Institutes of Health

Along with Full Contact Information for Each Agency

Edited by Wendy Wilcox. 698 pages. 1998. 0-7808-0220-9. $78.

"Recommended reference source."
— Booklist, American Library Association, Sep '98

"This consumer guide provides welcome assistance in navigating the maze of federal health agencies and their data on public health concerns."
— SciTech Book News, Sep '98

■

Reconstructive & Cosmetic Surgery Sourcebook

Basic Consumer Health Information on Cosmetic and Reconstructive Plastic Surgery, Including Statistical Information about Different Surgical Procedures, Things to Consider Prior to Surgery, Plastic Surgery Techniques and Tools, Emotional and Psychological Considerations, and Procedure-Specific Information

Along with a Glossary of Terms and a Listing of Resources for Additional Help and Information

Edited by M. Lisa Weatherford. 374 pages. 2001. 0-7808-0214-4. $78.

"Recommended for health science libraries that are open to the public, as well as hospital libraries that are open to the patients. This book is a good resource for the consumer interested in plastic surgery."
— E-Streams, Dec '01

"Recommended reference source."
— Booklist, American Library Association, July '01

Rehabilitation Sourcebook

Basic Consumer Health Information about Rehabilitation for People Recovering from Heart Surgery, Spinal Cord Injury, Stroke, Orthopedic Impairments, Amputation, Pulmonary Impairments, Traumatic Injury, and More, Including Physical Therapy, Occupational Therapy, Speech/ Language Therapy, Massage Therapy, Dance Therapy, Art Therapy, and Recreational Therapy

Along with Information on Assistive and Adaptive Devices, a Glossary, and Resources for Additional Help and Information

Edited by Dawn D. Matthews. 531 pages. 1999. 0-7808-0236-5. $78.

"This is an excellent resource for public library reference and health collections."
—American Reference Books Annual, 2001

"Recommended reference source."
—Booklist, American Library Association, May '00

■

Respiratory Diseases & Disorders Sourcebook

Basic Information about Respiratory Diseases and Disorders, Including Asthma, Cystic Fibrosis, Pneumonia, the Common Cold, Influenza, and Others, Featuring Facts about the Respiratory System, Statistical and Demographic Data, Treatments, Self-Help Management Suggestions, and Current Research Initiatives

Edited by Allan R. Cook and Peter D. Dresser. 771 pages. 1995. 0-7808-0037-0. $78.

"Designed for the layperson and for patients and their families coping with respiratory illness. . . . an extensive array of information on diagnosis, treatment, management, and prevention of respiratory illnesses for the general reader." *—Choice, Association of College and Research Libraries, Jun '96*

"A highly recommended text for all collections. It is a comforting reminder of the power of knowledge that good books carry between their covers."
—Academic Library Book Review, Spring '96

"A comprehensive collection of authoritative information presented in a nontechnical, humanitarian style for patients, families, and caregivers."
—Association of Operating Room Nurses, Sep/Oct '95

■

Sexually Transmitted Diseases Sourcebook, 1st Edition

Basic Information about Herpes, Chlamydia, Gonorrhea, Hepatitis, Nongonoccocal Urethritis, Pelvic Inflammatory Disease, Syphilis, AIDS, and More

Along with Current Data on Treatments and Preventions

Edited by Linda M. Ross. 550 pages. 1997. 0-7808-0217-9. $78.

Sexually Transmitted Diseases Sourcebook, 2nd Edition

Basic Consumer Health Information about Sexually Transmitted Diseases, Including Information on the Diagnosis and Treatment of Chlamydia, Gonorrhea, Hepatitis, Herpes, HIV, Mononucleosis, Syphilis, and Others

Along with Information on Prevention, Such as Condom Use, Vaccines, and STD Education; And Featuring a Section on Issues Related to Youth and Adolescents, a Glossary, and Resources for Additional Help and Information

Edited by Dawn D. Matthews. 538 pages. 2001. 0-7808-0249-7. $78.

"Every school and public library should have a copy of this comprehensive and user-friendly reference book."
—Choice, Association of College & Research Libraries, Sep '01

"This is a highly recommended book. This is an especially important book for all school and public libraries." *—AIDS Book Review Journal, Jul-Aug '01*

"Recommended reference source."
—Booklist, American Library Association, Apr '01

"Recommended pick both for specialty health library collections and any general consumer health reference collection." *—The Bookwatch, Apr '01*

■

Skin Disorders Sourcebook

Basic Information about Common Skin and Scalp Conditions Caused by Aging, Allergies, Immune Reactions, Sun Exposure, Infectious Organisms, Parasites, Cosmetics, and Skin Traumas, Including Abrasions, Cuts, and Pressure Sores

Along with Information on Prevention and Treatment

Edited by Allan R. Cook. 647 pages. 1997. 0-7808-0080-X. $78.

". . . comprehensive, easily read reference book."
—Doody's Health Sciences Book Reviews, Oct '97

***SEE ALSO** Burns Sourcebook*

■

Sleep Disorders Sourcebook

Basic Consumer Health Information about Sleep and Its Disorders, Including Insomnia, Sleepwalking, Sleep Apnea, Restless Leg Syndrome, and Narcolepsy

Along with Data about Shiftwork and Its Effects, Information on the Societal Costs of Sleep Deprivation, Descriptions of Treatment Options, a Glossary of Terms, and Resource Listings for Additional Help

Edited by Jenifer Swanson. 439 pages. 1998. 0-7808-0234-9. $78.

"This text will complement any home or medical library. It is user-friendly and ideal for the adult reader."
—American Reference Books Annual, 2000

"A useful resource that provides accurate, relevant, and accessible information on sleep to the general public. Health care providers who deal with sleep disorders patients may also find it helpful in being prepared to answer some of the questions patients ask."
— *Respiratory Care, Jul '99*

"Recommended reference source."
— *Booklist, American Library Association, Feb '99*

■

Sports Injuries Sourcebook

Basic Consumer Health Information about Common Sports Injuries, Prevention of Injury in Specific Sports, Tips for Training, and Rehabilitation from Injury

Along with Information about Special Concerns for Children, Young Girls in Athletic Training Programs, Senior Athletes, and Women Athletes, and a Directory of Resources for Further Help and Information

Edited by Heather E. Aldred. 624 pages. 1999. 0-7808-0218-7. $78.

"While this easy-to-read book is recommended for all libraries, it should prove to be especially useful for public, high school, and academic libraries; certainly it should be on the bookshelf of every school gymnasium."
— *E-Streams, Mar '00*

"Public libraries and undergraduate academic libraries will find this book useful for its nontechnical language."
— *American Reference Books Annual, 2000*

■

Stress-Related Disorders Sourcebook

Basic Consumer Health Information about Stress and Stress-Related Disorders, Including Stress Origins and Signals, Environmental Stress at Work and Home, Mental and Emotional Stress Associated with Depression, Post-Traumatic Stress Disorder, Panic Disorder, Suicide, and the Physical Effects of Stress on the Cardiovascular, Immune, and Nervous Systems

Along with Stress Management Techniques, a Glossary, and a Listing of Additional Resources

Edited by Joyce Brennfleck Shannon. 600 pages. 2002. 0-7808-0560-7. $78.

■

Substance Abuse Sourcebook

Basic Health-Related Information about the Abuse of Legal and Illegal Substances Such as Alcohol, Tobacco, Prescription Drugs, Marijuana, Cocaine, and Heroin; and Including Facts about Substance Abuse Prevention Strategies, Intervention Methods, Treatment and Recovery Programs, and a Section Addressing the Special Problems Related to Substance Abuse during Pregnancy

Edited by Karen Bellenir. 573 pages. 1996. 0-7808-0038-9. $78.

"A valuable addition to any health reference section. Highly recommended."
— *The Book Report, Mar/Apr '97*

"... a comprehensive collection of substance abuse information that's both highly readable and compact. Families and caregivers of substance abusers will find the information enlightening and helpful, while teachers, social workers and journalists should benefit from the concise format. Recommended."
— *Drug Abuse Update, Winter '96/'97*

SEE ALSO *Alcoholism Sourcebook, Drug Abuse Sourcebook*

■

Transplantation Sourcebook

Basic Consumer Health Information about Organ and Tissue Transplantation, Including Physical and Financial Preparations, Procedures and Issues Relating to Specific Solid Organ and Tissue Transplants, Rehabilitation, Pediatric Transplant Information, the Future of Transplantation, and Organ and Tissue Donation

Along with a Glossary and Listings of Additional Resources

Edited by Joyce Brennfleck Shannon. 628 pages. 2002. 0-7808-0322-1. $78.

■

Traveler's Health Sourcebook

Basic Consumer Health Information for Travelers, Including Physical and Medical Preparations, Transportation Health and Safety, Essential Information about Food and Water, Sun Exposure, Insect and Snake Bites, Camping and Wilderness Medicine, and Travel with Physical or Medical Disabilities

Along with International Travel Tips, Vaccination Recommendations, Geographical Health Issues, Disease Risks, a Glossary, and a Listing of Additional Resources

Edited by Joyce Brennfleck Shannon. 613 pages. 2000. 0-7808-0384-1. $78.

"Recommended reference source."
— *Booklist, American Library Association, Feb '01*

"This book is recommended for any public library, any travel collection, and especially any collection for the physically disabled."
— *American Reference Books Annual, 2001*

■

Women's Health Concerns Sourcebook

Basic Information about Health Issues That Affect Women, Featuring Facts about Menstruation and Other Gynecological Concerns, Including Endometriosis, Fibroids, Menopause, and Vaginitis; Reproductive Concerns, Including Birth Control, Infertility, and Abortion; and Facts about Additional Physical, Emotional, and Mental Health Concerns Prevalent among Women Such as Osteoporosis, Urinary Tract Disorders, Eating Disorders, and Depression

Along with Tips for Maintaining a Healthy Lifestyle

Edited by Heather E. Aldred. 567 pages. 1997. 0-7808-0219-5. $78.

"Handy compilation. There is an impressive range of diseases, devices, disorders, procedures, and other physical and emotional issues covered . . . well organized, illustrated, and indexed." —Choice, Association of College and Research Libraries, Jan '98

SEE ALSO Breast Cancer Sourcebook, Cancer Sourcebook for Women, 1st and 2nd Editions, Healthy Heart Sourcebook for Women, Osteoporosis Sourcebook

■

Workplace Health & Safety Sourcebook

Basic Consumer Health Information about Workplace Health and Safety, Including the Effect of Workplace Hazards on the Lungs, Skin, Heart, Ears, Eyes, Brain, Reproductive Organs, Musculoskeletal System, and Other Organs and Body Parts

Along with Information about Occupational Cancer, Personal Protective Equipment, Toxic and Hazardous Chemicals, Child Labor, Stress, and Workplace Violence

Edited by Chad T. Kimball. 626 pages. 2000. 0-7808-0231-4. $78.

"As a reference for the general public, this would be useful in any library." —E-Streams, Jun '01

"Provides helpful information for primary care physicians and other caregivers interested in occupational medicine. . . . General readers; professionals."
— Choice, Association of College & Research Libraries, May '01

"Recommended reference source."
— Booklist, American Library Association, Feb '01

"Highly recommended." — The Bookwatch, Jan '01

Worldwide Health Sourcebook

Basic Information about Global Health Issues, Including Malnutrition, Reproductive Health, Disease Dispersion and Prevention, Emerging Diseases, Risky Health Behaviors, and the Leading Causes of Death

Along with Global Health Concerns for Children, Women, and the Elderly, Mental Health Issues, Research and Technology Advancements, and Economic, Environmental, and Political Health Implications, a Glossary, and a Resource Listing for Additional Help and Information

Edited by Joyce Brennfleck Shannon. 614 pages. 2001. 0-7808-0330-2. $78.

"Named an Outstanding Academic Title."
—Choice, Association of College & Research Libraries, Jan '02

"Yet another handy but also unique compilation in the extensive Health Reference Series, this is a useful work because many of the international publications reprinted or excerpted are not readily available. Highly recommended."
—Choice, Association of College & Research Libraries, Nov '01

"Recommended reference source."
—Booklist, American Library Association, Oct '01

Health Reference Series